POSTERIOR CORTICAL ATROPHY

Dementia Guide for Doctors, Nurses, Patients, Families, Caregivers, & Medical Students

JERRY BELLER HEALTH RESEARCH
INSTITUTE

DEDICATION

To people living with Dementia and their loved ones.

CONTENTS

ACKNOWLEDGMENTS

Thanks to the American Academy of Neurology, Atlanta Center for Medical Research, Alzheimer's Association, Alzheimer's Disease Center, Alzheimer's Disease Center of Northwestern University, Alzheimer's Foundation of America, American Academy of Neurology, Association for Frontotemporal Degeneration, Australia Neurological Research, CDC, Department of Health and Human Services, Duke University Medical Center, Emory Hospital, Harvard Medical School, Johns Hopkins Medicine, Mayo Clinic, National Aphasia Association, National Institute of Neurological Disorders and Strokes, National Library of Medicine, National Institute on Aging, National Institutes of Health, Prince of Wales Medical Research Institute, *PubMed*, Stanford Library School of Medicine, Stanford Medicine, UCSF Department of Neurology, UCSF Memory and Aging Center, University of Cambridge Neurology Unit, World Health Organization (WHO), *Journal of American Medical Association* (JAMA), and several other organizations that provided information used for this book. Thanks to everybody who assisted this book in a variety of important ways, and everybody at Beller Health Research Institute. To my editor, John Briggs, who helps me improve every book. To all sources and for the photos. Most of all, thanks to my wife, Nicola Beller

FOREWORD

Before diving into the book's subject matter, let's discuss two related Dementia series:

- *2020 Dementia Overview* series
- *2020 Dementia Types, Symptoms, Stages, & Risk Factors* series

2020 Dementia Overview series is an extension of the medical groundbreaking *19 Dementia Types, Symptoms, Stages, & Risk Factors* series, the first covering all primary dementia types.

After spending decades building an audience in other genres, including nutrition, circumstances turned the world upside down. Doctors diagnosed my mother with Alzheimer's. The same doctors soon diagnosed my father with cancer. A few months later, my father's favorite brother and my closest uncle died.

Three consecutive hard blows blew the world beyond recognition.

Tough and decent as they come, dad insisted on taking care of my mother while fighting brain cancer. My brothers and sister-in-law did their share, but Dad cared for my mother for a long time while they worked. Dad proved what a remarkable and great man he was down the stretch but finally succumbed to brain cancer.

My brothers and sister-in-law did their best to take care of mom, but it came at a price. Caregiving for a dementia patient is an indescribable horror I would not wish on my worst enemy.

You must watch somebody you love wilt away, little by little until dementia wipes away huge chunks of their personality.

Living away, my wife and I visited when possible. We saw how mom deteriorated, but also the effect caregiving had on my father and brothers. It was like watching a train wreck over and over, each time getting worse and helpless to prevent it.

Watching Alzheimer's takedown, my strong-willed mother and others bruised my soul. My writing shifted initially to learn about Alzheimer's, but the more learned, the more I cringed.

The cold hard facts rendered me speechless. Over 5.8 million Americans, and 44 million people worldwide, suffer Alzheimer's. No cure. Just a devastating and expensive slow march towards an agonizing end.

Not content to kill, Alzheimer's tortured Mom for years before killing her. It robbed her memory and damaged her brain, where she repeated herself in a continuous loop, each time thinking she was saying it the first time. As the disease advanced, the neurological disorder destroyed her mind and body.

Seeing dementia take down that tough old bird rattled me. While I could not bring back my mother, I dedicate my life to researching and writing about dementia 8-12 hours per day, six or seven days per week.

I tackled Alzheimer's to learn everything I could about the brute and determine how I and others might prevent it and other noncommunicable diseases. Having written on nutrition and advocated health in Washington, I already had a clue but determined to figure out how to prevent Alzheimer's. But I needed to know more, much more, about this terrorizing neurological disorder.

I learned Alzheimer's was just one of over one-hundred neurological disorders causing dementia. When I searched for a book covering the primary dementias, none existed. Instead, I turned to individual books and again found no books written on several of the most frequent dementias.

In what on the one hand seems like yesterday and the other a lifetime ago, I set out several years ago to write a dementia book covering the 15 most prevalent dementia types. The first to do that, I next wrote books covering each of the 15 most prevalent dementias.

In 2020, I expanded the book covering 15 dementias to 19 dementia types. I also released books on each of the 19 dementias. While proud of these medical firsts, I do not take myself too seriously.

As one of the dozens of scientists, neurologists, researchers, and writers who devote their lives to fighting the war against dementia, I remain humble. I appreciate the individual and combined accomplishments of everybody else in the field.

Nor should any of us get cocky knowing we're losing the war. If we win the war during my lifetime, I will celebrate with hundreds of people worldwide who helped defeat the great beast of our day.

My two-book series break medical ground, and I consider major achievements but remain two among hundreds of significant contributions to the dementia field by people around the globe.

The series provides patients and loved ones a great resource for dementias not covered as extensive as Alzheimer's and the more prevalent types.

By covering the 19 most prevalent dementias, doctors, nurses, and medical professionals benefit from a series covering neurological disorders causing 99% of dementia. The series helps primary care physicians, providers, and nurses who struggle to diagnose dementias with overlapping symptoms.

The series is an organic, evolving work, and each book receives major annual updates. As science uncovers information, we add important data in new editions. We also polish each edition.

We describe the writing goal in three ways:

1. Simplify the language and make it easier for nonscientists to comprehend.
2. Honor the science and facts.
3. Document science and include citations for doctors,

nurses, medical researchers, students, and patients.

Our goal is to provide invaluable medical information for professionals, patients, loved ones, and caregivers.

I do not reinvent the wheel but accumulate the best research and teach our readers a better understanding of Alzheimer's and the other 18 primary dementia types.

Among the worst news is one of our loved ones has dementia. A killer disease with no cure frightens the bravest souls.

This medical condition destroys, not just the inflicted, but their loved ones. Besides the patient, nobody suffers more than voluntary caregivers. Watching a mother, father, brother, sister, wife, or husband suffering dementia brutalizes the soul.

I study dementia year around to write and release annual updates to honor people—including my mother—taken by Alzheimer's or one of the other primary dementias.

Modest book royalties are the only compensation, as I accept no money from corporations to promote their product. Nor do I have an ax to grind with anybody in the medical profession.

Having written 100 plus books over four decades, I am thankful to readers for collectively providing me a decent income. However, now in my sixties, I care little about riches and fame.

Who is the reading audience?

The audience falls into five categories.

Those Diagnosed with Dementia

If doctors diagnose you with dementia, my heart goes out to you. You're in for a long battle. Do yourself a favor and focus on slowing the disease and extending the quality of life. One word of caution, the books in this series speak to not only patients, but also families, doctors, students, nurses, and caregivers. Many of those diagnosed with dementia appreciate and benefit from the books, but some find some of the material too disturbing. I intend to write books exclusively for patients but must finish the work related to this series first. While there is not anything too shocking, I wrote the material for a wide audience, meaning I am not always speaking to patients specifically. I promise to personalize an edition for patients and loved ones after finishing this series. By shining a light on all 19 primary dementia types, I hope to help the medical community better distinguish and diagnose neurological disorders.

Loved Ones of Those Diagnosed

If doctors diagnose a loved one with dementia, he or she needs you more than ever. Depending on the type, dementia causes behavioral problems, memory issues, motor decline, and other psychological and physical disorders. The learning curve is steep and changes as one moves from one stage to the next. As with those with dementia, I warn families these books provide a technical overview, and the emphasis is not always on the emotional aspect. If you want to learn about dementias, this series is a great option. If you're looking more for emotional support, there are more appropriate books. I also plan to write a book specifically for families once fulfilling responsibilities for this series.

Medical Professionals

If you are a medical professional interested in studying the dementias, the series covers the dementias responsible for 99% of dementia. While neurologists probably already know the 19 primary dementias, the books provide a quick overview and reference for primary care physicians, nurses, other medical professionals, and students. I also include citations so you can continue your investigation beyond the book's scope.

Volunteer & Professional Caregivers

If you are a dementia caregiver, you are also in for a long, difficult march. Dementia patients demand 24/7 care in later stages, requiring help to go to the bathroom, bathing, and other basic daily functions. While this series is not written solely for caregiving, caregivers benefit by gaining a better understanding of each dementia, their symptoms, and progression.

Anybody Wanting to Learn About A Disease That Strikes 1 Of 6 Americans, And 1 Of 3 Seniors

The series benefits anybody who wants to gain an intermediate understanding of the 19 dementias.

Series' First Lesson

Doctors, like teachers, are part of a sacred profession. **Nothing I say or write replaces your need for a competent doctor!** Nor does any criticism of the profession diminish my respect and admiration for the best.

I detest the worst teachers who fail students and society but love and respect the best. Society would crumble without the most devoted and competent teachers.

Similar, I abhor incompetent, greedy doctors who fail patients and society, but love and respect the best.

The profession must weed out incompetent, uncaring, corrupt doctors, and medical personnel. Every profession has a percentage of bad apples, but within the medical profession, they are cancerous!

Nothing good I write about the medical profession includes incompetent, uncaring doctors, researchers, nurses, etc. And nothing bad I write targets the best.

The series criticizes the profession when deserved, but the first lesson in this series: **Find a competent doctor!** If you have one, count your blessings. If not, find one.

Just as one can learn outside the classroom, we live in a blessed age where medical information is available for anybody on the internet. Such information serves us well, but do not—for a minute-think it replaces the need for a competent, devoted doctor.

The Wrong Doctors

Let me begin this section by saying I love and respect quality doctors, nurses, researchers, and medical professionals from the bottom of my heart and the fullness of my mind.

However, this section is not about what's right in the medical profession.

Glorified idiots, bad doctors are dangerous parasites who dishonor a noble profession. Smart enough to finish medical school, but greedy or flawed beyond redemption, they are like priests working for the devil. Among the worse members of society are doctors motivated by greed or limited by incompetence. Walking parasites!

The Wrong Doctors + Big Pharm + Big Insurance + Big Hospital = Expensive & Inadequate Health Care

Over the past few decades, Big pharmaceuticals, Big Insurance, and their political puppets appointed doctors sanctioned drug dealers. Entrusting the worse doctors with such powers produces little or no better results than assigning the task to a thug on the worst corner in America.

The worst doctors who hand out drugs like candy serve nobody's purpose but their own and Big Pharm.

Not an indictment of the entire profession, but unfortunately, Big Insurance dictates the typical office visit includes a quick examination and one or more prescriptions. The approach is not based on good science and runs counter to everything science teaches us.

What About Some Tough Love?

The one thing people today do not want is what we often need most, tough love. People want everything sugarcoated and easy.

The problem is most of the time; life is neither sweet nor easy.

What patients need much of the time is not an alleged "magic pill," but instead tough love. Doctors must learn nutrition and teach patients to eat healthier, exercise more, and get 7-8 hours of sleep per night. Like it or not, this is part of modern medicine. Showing up and passing out pills all day is not preventing Alzheimer's and other dementias, nor curing them.

Medical professionals must lead by example and embrace the science of nutrition, exercise, and sleep. If a healthy diet and exercise are the two cornerstones to health, the third is sleep.

The average person needs few or no drugs if they practice healthy habits.

Any doctor who does not vigorously advocate a balanced whole food diet, exercise most days of the week, and 7-8 hours' sleep per night neglects their duty and

Instead, too many doctors ignore the three cornerstones of health and are content to write their patients unnecessary and potentially dangerous prescriptions for the rest of their lives. 100% emphasis on treating symptoms with drugs, which often require more drugs to counter the side effects, is producing disastrous results. To be the best doctor, one must also emphasize prevention.

Failed Drug Trials

None of the drug trials have produced even one drug that cures Alzheimer's and other dementias. While science has failed to produce any effective dementia drugs, scientific studies prove we can do much by practicing healthy habits to slow or reduce our dementia risk.

The Medical Profession Must Think Outside The Box

The hopeless circle of failed drug trials demands we think outside the box or, as neurologist David Perlmutter advocates, expand the box. He and other neurologists deserve credit for recognizing medicine is failing the dementia war and rocking the boat of conventional wisdom. I must not agree with every point "maverick" neurologists like David Perlmutter, Dale Bredesen, and Deepak Chopra make to respect them for turning conventional wisdom on its head.

Conventional wisdom is losing the Alzheimer's and dementia war!

Not Anti-doctors or Anti-drugs

I am not anti-doctors or anti-drugs and do not understand those who insist neither are needed. I revere competent doctors who practice and advocate the three cornerstones of health. I also recognize the polio vaccine and many other drugs as nothing short of miraculous.

But, my love for what is right about the medical profession will not silence me about what is wrong. And, pretending drugs are the answer to defeating Alzheimer's or dementia is a colossal failure.

You cannot "**do no harm**" and write prescription drugs at the volume of the average doctor.

Choose A Doctor with The Same Care As You Do A Spouse

Find a competent, dedicated, caring, experienced, informed, ethical doctor who listens and respects your opinion, and writes prescriptions as a LAST RESORT.

Without the right doctor, you are at the mercy of a profit-oriented health system that seldom puts the patient's interests first, second, or third.

Nothing I say or write in these books or elsewhere means you should not see a doctor, stop taking your medication, or otherwise undermine the medical profession's ability to diagnose and treat any medical symptoms you might experience.

Find a good doctor you trust with your life and ask him or her pointed questions concerning your health and any treatment they recommend.

Outside the Bubble

I challenge the medical profession where necessary, just as I criticize Congress and the United States government for their mistakes or shortcomings. My brief career as a Congressional staffer taught me how difficult it is to maintain one's focus inside the bubble.

Seeing the big picture is no less challenging inside the medical bubble motivated by profit.

Profiteers fund too many studies to promote their product or discredit somebody else's. Blatant self-interests taint studies and confuse the public. Such contradictory studies confuse and make it impossible for the average person to understand which studies to believe.

I respect ethical, competent, dedicated, and hardworking nurses, doctors, and other medical personnel. As much as I criticize what is wrong within the profession, I cannot praise the majority of medical professionals often enough. Getting quality medical care when we need it is one of life's greatest blessings.

Nor do I object to medical-related businesses making a reasonable profit in return for needed medical supplies and services.

Nor should any competent and ethical medical professionals object to anybody challenging medical incompetence and profiteers.

Trust Thy Doctor

The right doctor does not discriminate between physical and mental diseases, so hold back nothing if you or a loved one exhibits symptoms.

If you lack the right doctor, find the right one. Outside you and the daily habits you establish, nobody is more important than your doctor for your health. You must be able to tell him or her medical information you might be reluctant to tell your closest confidant in life.

Remember, doctors too often misdiagnose dementia. Once the symptoms of these deadly dementias set in, you need to see your doctor, provide them with all the information about your problem, and help the specialists reach the correct diagnosis.

Because no tests exist for most dementias, doctors order tests and go through a process of elimination until reaching a diagnosis based on the symptoms you report. The more information you provide, the better the chance of a quick and accurate diagnosis.

Adopt healthy lifestyle choices to prevent dementia when possible, but the next best option is to diagnose it early, to confront it head-on, and take steps to slow the disease. Once dementia hits, it's often possible to postpone the advanced stages. If you've seen a loved one inflicted with dementia, you understand how precious a year, a month, a week, or day is once the storm aims at you or a loved one.

Prolonging life in late-stage dementia without a cure amounts to cruel and unusual punishment, but patients, families, and doctors must do everything possible to extend quality of life while possible.

Make certain you have a doctor who believes in prevention and natural cures, but also remember you need their expertise concerning the best that modern medicine offers.

Be Your Nurse!

If you have a loved one, be each other's nurse. If not, be your nurse.

It's more important than ever for you to monitor your blood pressure and make notes of health issues as they arise. We don't go to the doctor every time we develop a symptom or don't feel well, but it's important to keep a medical journal. Write an outline of the problems you experience between visits.

Too often, we march into the physician's office and don't provide a full or accurate representation of our problem. For instance, if you track your blood pressure, you can furnish a

11

pattern rather than a onetime reading. You can also perhaps attribute pikes in your blood pressure to stress taking place in your life.

You should also track other symptoms. Providing thorough information helps doctors eliminate multiple diseases with similar symptoms. When you document all or most of the symptoms that have led to the visit, you provide a competent doctor a clearer picture to develop a hypothesis. These previous unrelated symptoms might help your physician make more sense of what prompted the appointment.

Otherwise, your physician might order the wrong tests or prescribe the wrong drugs. For issues of the brain, you can't be shy or embarrassed about providing your physician with a full portrayal of your problems and symptoms.

Although still stigmatized in some circles, mental illnesses are just as real, and the sufferers are no more the blame, than physical disorders. While we must do everything in our power to avoid or slow mental or physical maladies, the last thing we need to do is embarrass those who are already suffering.

Two Dementia Series

The laborious task to document the primary dementias began as a fifty-page Alzheimer's overview. Two editions later, the 50-page Alzheimer's book turned into 400 pages.

One of the first lessons taught Alzheimer's is only one of the hundreds of diseases responsible for dementia. With inadequate testing, similar symptoms, and other handicaps, the medical community often misdiagnoses the other dementias for Alzheimer's.

My focus broadened from Alzheimer's to a dozen dementias. The only way to make any sense of Alzheimer's or dementia was to study all the primary dementias.

I worked with several neurologists and researchers over the next couple of years and hit every medical library I could hit in person or available online.

After an extensive review, I wrote the first book covering the 15 most prevalent dementia types, which provided the groundwork for two updated dementia series.

The associated *Dementia Types, Symptoms, Stages, & Risk Factors, series* expands the collection by adding amyotrophic lateral sclerosis (ALS), early-onset Alzheimer's disease, amyotrophic lateral sclerosis, corticobasal syndrome, and progressive supranuclear palsy.

Two Dementia Series

Not counting mixed dementia, there are nineteen primary dementia types, which two groundbreaking series covers.

Dementia Types, Symptoms, Stages, & Risk Factors series

1. _Dementia with Lewy Bodies_
2. _Parkinson's Disease Dementia_
3. Corticobasal Syndrome
4. Typical Alzheimer's Disease
5. _Posterior Cortical Atrophy_
6. _Down Syndrome with Alzheimer's_
7. _Limbic-predominant Age-related TDP-43 Encephalopathy (LATE)_
8. Early-onset Alzheimer's
9. _Behavioral Variant Frontotemporal Dementia_
10. Progressive Supranuclear Palsy
11. _Nonfluent Primary Progressive Aphasia_
12. Logopenic Progressive Aphasia
13. _Cortical Vascular Dementia_
14. _Binswanger Disease_
15. _Normal Pressure Hydrocephalus_
16. _Huntington's Disease_
17. _Korsakoff Syndrome_
18. _Creutzfeldt-Jakob Disease_
19. Amyotrophic Lateral Sclerosis

*Not a dementia type, but a combination, mixed dementia is the 20th category important in dementia discussions.

Any disease leading to associated symptoms is a dementia type. The series breaks medical ground by covering the dementias responsible for over 99% of dementia cases.

Dementia Overview Series

The second series focuses on all the primary dementia types or breaks them down as groups.

2020 Dementia Overview Series

1. Dementia Types, Symptoms, & Stages
2. *Lewy Body/Parkinsonism Dementias*
3. *Vascular Dementia*
4. *Frontotemporal Dementia (FTD)*
5. Alzheimer's Related Dementias
6. *Prevent or Slow Dementia*

The Best Science in Everyday Language

The text in both series contains American, Australian, British, and other English. I write in American English, but the research comes from the best studies worldwide. Quotes from the UK, Australia, and other English-speaking countries depend on the local dialect. For integrity, I do not edit quotes.

The books include facts and science as they exist. As much as possible, we replace medical jargon with everyday language.

Having explained the series, let's discuss dementia.

I. DEMENTIA

In this section, we discuss dementia.

Dementia is not a disease but a medical condition. Hundreds of diseases and disorders lead to dementia, but percentage-wise, almost all dementia falls under 19 primary dementia categories.

This series is the first to cover all 19 primary dementia types.

In this chapter, we answer the following questions:

- What is dementia?
- What are the 19 primary dementias?
- How prevalent is dementia?
- Who is most likely to get dementia?
- What are the financial costs to individuals, the U.S., and worldwide?

Once we answer these questions and provide a dementia overview, we turn our attention to the subject matter for the rest of the book.

Let's begin by answering the question: What is dementia?

Chapter 1: WHAT IS DEMENTIA?

For centuries, when one got dementia, people described the person in terms like "gone mad," or "lost their mind," or "crazy," or another derogatory term that missed the mark.

While most dementia types attack cognitive skills and cause behavioral disorders, the person is no less a victim than a cancer patient.

Whereas cancer attacks cells and organs, dementia destroys brain neurons.

The brain is complex. One-hundred billion neurons use over 100 trillion synapses and about 100 neurotransmitters to send all the signals to other parts of the brain, organs, and parts throughout the body, allowing us to think, reason, walk, talk, breathe, and do all that makes us human.

When fed, protected, and healthy, neurons perform magic.

The different dementias attack the brain and destroy the communication network responsible for everything our body does. By attacking different parts of the brain, the dementia types cause different disorders.

Let's see how some of the most prestigious American and global medical organizations define Dementia.

Alzheimer's Association Definition

Let's begin with the Alzheimer's Association:

Dementia is an overall term for diseases and conditions characterized by a decline in memory, language, problem-solving, and other thinking skills that affect a person's ability to perform everyday activities. Memory loss is an example. Alzheimer's is the most common cause of dementia[1].

Dementia is to Alzheimer's, dementia with Lewy bodies,

Parkinson's dementia, vascular and the other dementia types what Asia is to China, India, North Korea, South Korea, and the rest of Asia. Alzheimer's is the most prevalent dementia, but each type devastates, and most are death sentences.

Let's turn to the National Institute on Aging (NIH) and see how they define dementia.

National Institute on Aging (NIH)

The National Institute on Aging (NIH) funds many studies and provides researchers invaluable data. How do they define dementia?

> *Dementia is the loss of cognitive functioning — thinking, remembering, and reasoning — and behavioral abilities to such an extent that it interferes with a person's daily life and activities. These functions include memory, language skills, visual perception, problem-solving, self-management, and the ability to focus and pay attention. Some people with dementia cannot control their emotions, and their personalities may change. Dementia ranges in severity from the mildest stage, when it is just beginning to affect a person's functioning, to the most severe stage, when the person must depend completely on others for basic activities of living[2].*

One of the most important things a person and their loved ones can do when diagnosed with dementia; enjoy what quality time remains.

Early diagnosis, medication, and lifestyle changes can slow the disease and extend quality life. From the point of diagnosis, make the most of each good day or moment.

Let's see how the international community defines dementia.

Alzheimer's Society UK

The Alzheimer's Society is perhaps the UK's most

prestigious Alzheimer's organization. They define dementia:

The word 'dementia' describes a set of symptoms that may include memory loss and difficulties with thinking, problem-solving or language. These changes are often small to start with, but for someone with dementia they have become severe enough to affect daily life. A person with dementia may also experience changes in their mood or behaviour[3].

Let's see how the World Health Organization (WHO) defines dementia.

World Health Organization (WHO)

The World Health Organization (WHO) works with global medical organizations and provides researchers a wealth of information. How does WHO define dementia?

Dementia is a syndrome – usually of a chronic or progressive nature – in which there is deterioration in cognitive function (i.e. the ability to process thought) beyond what might be expected from normal ageing. It affects memory, thinking, orientation, comprehension, calculation, learning capacity, language, and judgement. Consciousness is not affected. The impairment in cognitive function is commonly accompanied, and occasionally preceded, by deterioration in emotional control, social behaviour, or motivation[4].

The four organizations provide similar definitions, each emphasizing different points, but none contradicting the others.

Each organization confirms dementia is a broad neurological disorder. Hundreds of pathologies such as Alzheimer's leads to dementia, but 19 primary types cause about 99% of dementia cases. Dementia attacks the brain and causes memory decline, behavior disorders, motor decline, language deterioration, and most types are incurable.

If doctors diagnose you with dementia, you must get past the shock. Time is moving against you, so make the most of it.

As the Alzheimer's Society points out, the symptoms are minor in the beginning. Get your affairs in order, enjoy loved ones, and take part in as many activities as you desire and are able. To some extent, this is your farewell tour. Take advantage!

The disease will stop you or a loved one later, so do not stop living your life in the early stages.

Let's next examine the 19 primary dementia types.

Chapter 2: WHAT ARE THE 19 PRIMARY DEMENTIAS?

Hundreds of medical conditions lead to dementia, but 19 causes up to 99% of cases.

Each dementia type is devastating, most are fatal, and the first symptoms to death is a challenging, heartbreaking, soul-crushing experience. Dementia robs the personalities and functionality of marvelous people a little at a time until they no longer resemble the person they've always been.

19 Dementia Types

This chapter divides the 19 primary dementias into six categories. The first group includes dementias related to Lewy body or Parkinsonism dementia. The second consists of Alzheimer's-related dementia. In the third, we focus on primary progressive aphasia dementias. The fourth contains vascular dementias. The fifth category encompasses the remaining dementias and is called *other dementias.*

Lewy Body/Parkinsonism Related Dementias

1. *Dementia with Lewy Bodies*
2. *Parkinson's Disease Dementia*
3. Corticobasal Syndrome

Alzheimer's Related Dementias

4. Typical Alzheimer's Disease
5. *Posterior Cortical Atrophy*
6. *Down Syndrome with Alzheimer's*
7. *Limbic-predominant Age-related TDP-43 Encephalopathy (LATE)*
8. Early-onset Alzheimer's

Frontotemporal Lobar Degeneration Related Dementias

9. *Behavioral Variant Frontotemporal Dementia*
10. Progressive Supranuclear Palsy

Primary Progressive Aphasia Related Dementias

11. *Nonfluent Primary Progressive Aphasia (nfvPPA)*
12. Logopenic Progressive Aphasia (LPA)

Vascular Dementia

13. *Cortical Vascular Dementia*
14. *Binswanger Disease*

Other Dementias

15. *Normal Pressure Hydrocephalus*
16. *Huntington's Disease*
17. *Korsakoff Syndrome*
18. *Creutzfeldt-Jakob Disease*
19. Amyotrophic Lateral Sclerosis

Chapter 3: WHO IS MOST LIKELY TO GET DEMENTIA?

In this chapter, we explore who is most likely to get dementia. Most know people with dementia are old, but some people are born with dementia, others get it as infants, and the disease attacks people in every age group.

There are risk factors that affect everybody. Examples include a poor diet, lack of exercise, diabetes, obesity, high blood pressure, and factors under and beyond our control.

In this chapter, we focus on risk factors affecting specific groups of people who suffer higher rates.

The research pointed to age, race, and sex, where dementia seems to discriminate. Let's review the science for each.

Age

Age is the obvious risk factor. We know because of science and our observations.

So associated with the elderly, many believe dementia only strikes older people. However, dementia strikes all ages and demographics, including newborns and infants.

According to Stanford University Medical School, "The risk of Alzheimer's disease, vascular dementia, and several other dementias goes up significantly with advancing age[5]."

None of us enjoy aging. We must work harder and harder to slow aging, and no matter how well we do, none of us will make it much past 100 years. The better we take care of ourselves, the higher chance we have of living a quality life into our eighties or nineties.

Remember, aging does not destroy our cognitive abilities. Bad habits do! I stress this point because each of us can slow the aging process through healthy habits.

As people age, however, our dementia risks increase.

A Journal of Neurology, Neurosurgery, & Psychiatry study

concluded[6]:

> *In the age group 65–69 years, there are more than two new cases per 1000 persons every year. This number increases almost exponentially with increasing age, until over the age of 90 years, out of 1000 persons, 70 new cases of dementia can be expected every year.*

As we stress in our book on prevention, there is actual age and real age. We determine one's actual age by the day and year born, whereas weight, blood pressure, blood sugar, cholesterol, diet, how often you work out, and several other important factors govern our real age.

Unless genes or an accident prevents us, our real age should be lower than our actual age. Those who practice bad habits, however, raise their real age ten years or more than their actual age.

When our real age is lower than our actual age, we lower our risks for dementia and other diseases. When our real age is higher than our actual age, we increase risks for dementia, heart disease, cancer, and all major diseases.

Let's next review if race plays a role in dementia.

Race

African Americans and blacks in western countries suffer more than their share of racism.

The United States has abused too many citizens since its creation, but none more than Native Americans and African Americans.

But, does dementia also discriminate against them?

According to AARP, African Americans are 64% more likely to get dementia than non-Hispanic whites[7].

Kaiser Permanente Study

Researchers in another study examined data from 274,000

Kaiser Permanente patients over 14 years. They found the highest rate of dementia for African Americans and Native Americans[8].

Dementia Risk Per 1,000 People

- 27 African Americans
- 22 Native Americans
- 20 Latinos and Pacific Islanders
- 19 White Americans
- 15 Asian-Americans

Does dementia love Asian and European-Americans and hate African and Native-Americans?

Dementia is as evil as the worst bigot, but dementia is not a bigot.

African Americans experience higher rates of diabetes. African Americans and Native Americans suffer a higher level of stress, poverty, and disenfranchisement. Both cultures also struggle with their people's history in European-America and endure a greater level of bigotry and more obstacles to succeeding in modern America.

On the flip side, Asian Americans and whites have lower obesity and diabetes rates, eat a more balanced diet, faceless bigotry, are more affluent, educated, and successful in modern America.

We need more studies to confirm the exact causes of higher dementia incidence in the African and Native American populations. Higher stress and diabetes in their communities are prime suspects.

Jennifer Manly, Columbia University, Taub Institute for Research on Alzheimer's disease, and Aging Brain spoke to Reuters about the inequities.

There are huge disparities in dementia that are confronting this nation and this will translate into an enormous burden on families if

*we don't address this. We need to prioritize
research that uncovers the reasons for these
disparities and more research should include
racially and ethnically diverse people[9].*

Are African British at a greater risk for Dementia?

In the United Kingdom, black women are 25% more likely than white women, and black men 28% more likely than white men to get dementia[10].

Reluctance to Take Part in Dementia Studies

African Americans and Native Americans are also less trustful of studies. Too often in the past, a bigoted establishment treated African Americans and Native Americans like lab rats.

The awful past makes the average African American reluctant to take part in studies that might help us figure out how to lower the rates.

Native Americans are also distrustful of the United States government and the "white man's studies," as one group from the Cherokee Reservation in North Carolina told me.

I understand both ethnic groups' skepticism. As somebody with ancestors who died and survived the Trail of Tears, and who married a black woman (30+ years), nobody must convince me of the tainted American history. I have read about the past and viewed enough with my own eyes to know the sins of America's past, either haunt or still torment today.

But, the Studies are Necessary!

I call on African Americans and Native Americans to take part in dementia studies. The studies today have greater safeguards than the past and face much more scrutiny.

Dementia is a death sentence!

Worse than the average killer, never content to kill and move on, dementia is a sadist. Dementia destroys the mind and body, little by little, robbing one's personality, dignity, mind, body, and everything that makes a person unique.

If African Americans and Native Americans refuse to participate in dementia studies, fatal neurological disorders will continue to strike them worse than other ethnic groups.

Please consider two facts.

If you do not have dementia, researchers do not subject you to drug trials but accumulate data to determine which habits increase and decrease one's risks.

If doctors diagnose you with dementia, trials represent your last best chance to win what is otherwise a losing battle.

What Role does Poverty Play?

Although not listed as a dementia risk factor, poverty increases one's risk for almost every significant disease. Those at the bottom must worry where the next meal is coming, if somebody might mug (or kill) them when leaving the house, and a laundry list of stress the average citizen seems oblivious.

Beller Health calls for more research to determine if Native American, African American, and African British citizens have higher dementia rates as a general population, or if poverty drives these numbers. We need to know whether the number also applies to middle-and upper-class African Americans and Native Americans who eat healthily, exercise, do not abuse alcohol, avoid tobacco, and do not abuse prescription or illicit drugs.

Native American, African American, and African British citizens suffer a higher percentage of poverty than other demographics in the US and UK.

Rather than race, such factors as poverty, bigotry, and lack of opportunities might drive these numbers.

I reached out to several organizations, including the VA, to conduct a large-scale study to determine what role poverty plays in dementia. Most organizations greeted my request with enthusiasm, and I hope one or more soon back the study.

All we know for certain is poverty in the industrial world causes a much greater level of stress and other hardships than the rest of the population. WHO reported that about 60% of dementia cases occur in the poorest half of countries[11].

Age and ethnicity are dementia risk factors. What about sex?

Sex

Dementia strikes older people, African Americans, Native Americans, and African British in greater numbers than the rest of the population. Does one's gender increase or decrease one's odds?

How Many Women have Dementia?

According to the Alzheimer's Association, women represent two-thirds of people living with Alzheimer's, and 13 million women suffer dementia or are caring for somebody who does[12].

Of the 820,000 people living with dementia in the UK, females account for 61 percent[13].

Of the 50 million people living with dementia worldwide[14], women represent 65 percent[15].

Key points:

- Women represent two-thirds of Alzheimer's cases.
- Females account for 65% of dementia cases.

Is dementia just another woman-hating predator?

Does Alzheimer's & Most Dementia Strike Women in Greater Numbers?

While the two key numbers suggest dementia is a rampaging woman-abusing murderer, the answer is not so simple.

While women represent two-thirds of Alzheimer's cases and 65% of dementia cases, there are 19 primary dementia types.

Some dementias attack men in greater numbers and much harder than females. The dementias we know attack men in greater ratios include[16]:

- Parkinson's dementia (Lewy body dementia)
- Dementia with Lewy bodies (Lewy body dementia)
- Post-Stroke dementia (Vascular dementia)

- Multi-infarct dementia (Vascular dementia)
- Binswanger Disease(Vascular dementia)
- Normal pressure hydrocephalus
- Behavioral variant frontotemporal dementia
- Primary Progressive Aphasia (Frontotemporal dementia)
- Chronic traumatic encephalopathy
- HIV-related cognitive impairment
- Amyotrophic lateral sclerosis

From the data about the 19 primary dementias, at least eleven attack men in greater numbers. Data is not available for Creutzfeldt-Jakob disease, Wernicke-Korsakoff Syndrome, LATE, and Down syndrome with Alzheimer's disease. The remaining dementias strike both genders in similar numbers. When the authorities release more information, we will update this section.

If a minimum of 11 of 19 dementia types strike men in greater numbers than women, how can 68% of people living with dementia be women?

Alzheimer's accounts for 60-80% of dementia, and two-thirds of people with Alzheimer's are women.

When we say dementia attacks, women, 65% to 35% men, we distort the picture. I call on the medical community to provide greater clarity. More precise, we should warn women to represent two-thirds of total Alzheimer's cases, but stress a minimum of 11 of 19 dementia types strike men in greater numbers.

Treating dementia and Alzheimer's as interchangeable terms is misleading. There are 19 primary dementias and 11 or more attack men in greater numbers. If we exclude Alzheimer's and focus on the other 18 primary dementia types, they attack men by far greater percentages.

With that stipulation, let's explore why Alzheimer's and some dementias attack women more than men.

Why Does Alzheimer's & Dementia Strike Women in Greater Numbers Than Men?

In part, unique burdens & responsibilities explain the disparity.

Women still fight today for equality. Like Native Americans, African Americans, and African British, the average woman carries burdens; the average man is clueless.

To be a woman, one fights for equality from birth in a "man's world," as the song and tradition attest. Among things unique to women:

- Menstrual cycles (ranging from mild to horrendous)
- Childbirth
- Menopause

Being a guy is also difficult, but there's no denying women are born with unique responsibilities and burdens.

As an aunt once retorted, if they live long enough, every woman suffers menstrual cycles until menopause "tortures it out."

Women Live Longer

Women outlive men in the United States and worldwide.

Worldwide, the average man lives to age 69.8, while the average woman lives 74.2 years[17]. These are the average numbers, so they fluctuate from region to region and country to country.

Let's see how these numbers compare to the United States.

American Comparisons

The CDC reports the average American male lives 76 years, compared to the average American woman who lives 81 years[18].

Why Do Women Live Longer Than Men?

Although women live longer, this might result because

more men abuse alcohol, tobacco, and drugs, get less sleep, work in more hazardous jobs, suffer greater casualties in war, and take unnecessary risks.

The lead author of a study published in the *British Medical Journal*, Australian neuropsychiatrist Richard Cibulskis, confirmed some of my suspicions.

> *Men are much more likely to die from preventable and treatable non-communicable diseases, such as {ischemic} heart disease and lung cancer, and road traffic accidents[19].*

Global population expert, Dr. Perminder Sachdev, confirmed my other suspicions in an interview with *Time*.

"Men are more likely to smoke, drink excessively and be overweight," Sachdev said. "They are also less likely to seek medical help early, and, if diagnosed with a disease, they are more likely to be non-adherent to treatment." Sachdev also pointed out, "men are more likely to take life-threatening risks and to die in car accidents, brawls or gunfights[20]."

Although nature perhaps installed a natural order to preserve the female population, men's reckless nature might account for the five years difference in life expectancy between the genders.

It will interest to see if the numbers change as more women become more like men. Women are assuming greater roles in war, law enforcement, and other areas where even men with healthy habits have fallen. As the societal lines between men and women blur, the difference in life expectancy should fall.

In all honorable fields of life, women should go for it. Never has there been a better time to prove the equality of the sexes.

As far as men's bad habits, my hope is women continue to show better judgment and exercise greater restraint. Women will never prove their equality by emulating men's worse habits or trying to outdo us in the stupid department.

The best men and women rise on similar foundations. However, the worst men and women also share a foundation.

My hope for humans getting our act together soon hinges on the average woman being better than the average man.

Love yourselves for your unique feminine qualities. Be equal, but please do not confuse out-drinking, out-smoking, out-drugging, acting more reckless, and stupid than men with being equal. We need fewer men like that, not more women!

Chapter 4: DEMENTIA COSTS & PREVALENCE

In this chapter, we review dementia prevalence and costs to governments, the world, caregivers, and patients.

How Many People Worldwide Suffer Dementia?

According to the World Health Organization (WHO), over 50 million people suffer dementia worldwide, with 10 million new cases each year[21].

How Many Americans Have Dementia?

In the United States, 5.8 million Americans live with dementia[22], with Alzheimer's representing 70% of cases.

Let's check the UK dementia numbers.

How Many People In The UK Have Dementia?

According to the Alzheimer's Society, 850,000 people in the UK live with dementia[23].

Alzheimer's Society reports that about 70% of those living in UK care homes suffer dementia.

The numbers show Americans, British, and global citizens suffering high rates of dementia. Let's see which countries' dementia strikes the hardest.

Which Countries Have The Highest Dementia Rate?

Per World Atlas, the following ten countries suffer the highest dementia rate of deaths per 100,000 people[24]:

1. Finland
2. USA
3. Canada
4. Iceland
5. Sweden
6. Switzerland
7. Norway
8. Denmark
9. The Netherlands
10. Belgium

As we review the list, per population, dementia strikes Americans in greater numbers than any country but Finland.

Why?

There are several explanations:

- Over two-thirds of Americans are obese or overweight.
- The other countries on the list also suffer higher obesity levels than most countries not on the list.
- Because of weight issues, the countries in question suffer high rates of diabetes and high blood pressure, both dementia risk factors.
- Americans consume more prescription drugs than people worldwide. While there is no data to confirm, I suspect the other countries on the list also have greater access and use more prescription drugs than poorer countries.
- They load the western diet with salt, sugar, and

white processed flours.

- The average person in western countries lives longer than those in poorer nations.
- We will add other factors once data becomes available.
- People live longer in these countries than most not on the list (the older one lives, the greater the dementia risk)

Another explanation is more misdiagnosis and no-diagnosis in poorer countries around the world. Obesity and other risk factors are also less of a problem in developing countries.

I recommend global researchers compare the ten countries on this list. By viewing the similarities between the ten, we might better pinpoint the cause for Alzheimer's and the other dementias.

If we can figure out what the citizens from the ten nations are doing wrong, we can find the cause and means of preventing dementia. While I pointed to some of the most obvious risk factors, the most important common risk factor from the ten nations might be something unexpected.

Let's now examine dementia costs.

Dementia Costs

In this chapter, we analyze dementia costs. We examine the United States and global costs, then provide estimated costs per family.

What Does Dementia Cost the United States?

More than the entire economies of Finland and 166 other countries, dementia costs the United States $277 billion per year.

What Does Dementia Cost Worldwide?

Getting credible global numbers proves difficult, if not impossible, in any medical research. Often, the best source is the World Health Organization (WHO). They collect data from around the world and are an essential source for medical researchers.

Getting accurate dementia numbers in richer countries is difficult. In the United States and the UK, black people hesitate to take part in dementia studies or to seek medical attention for symptoms.

In richer countries, there are still too many misdiagnoses.

Thus, if we cannot get ironclad numbers in the United States, the United Kingdom, and the industrial nations, the task proves even more difficult for developing countries.

If the United States and the United Kingdom have difficulty convincing black citizens to seek medical attention for dementia symptoms, the third world faces even greater obstacles.

In the third world, most areas do well to offer their citizens basic medical care. With no urine or blood test, many regions lack resources for CAT scans, MRIs, and other expensive imaging equipment to make a diagnosis.

Without urine or blood tests, diagnosing dementia costs more than low-income people with inadequate or no insurance can afford in the richest countries.

In the United States and industrial nations, doctors often misdiagnose the other 19 primary dementias for Alzheimer's or each other.

Expecting doctors in many third world nations to diagnose dementia with inferior or no equipment is to expect miracles. If it overwhelms medical professionals in the wealthier nations, we often expect third world doctors to perform miracles. What amazes is they often do!

However, no matter how good a job the average third world doctor does treating typical medical conditions, even if trained, it does not equip them to diagnose dementia early, if at all. My comments are not criticism.

The average doctor's job is not to diagnose or treat dementia, but they must recognize symptoms and refer the patient to neurologists. Primary care physicians are the first line of defense.

North, south, east, west, dementia overwhelms the medical community.

Having discussed the limitations, let's examine the data. While the numbers are ballpark figures, landing in the park is the keystone to estimation. In most cases, the real numbers are much higher.

According to the *World Alzheimer's Report,* global dementia costs a minimum of $1 trillion per year, and experts predict it will reach $2 trillion by 2030 if we find no cure[25].

Authorities should release new numbers over the next year, and we will update this section.

The *Alzheimer's Report* global cost estimations do not include informal care costs; another reason we consider the estimates conservative.

The Alzheimer's Report concluded:

> *Direct medical care costs account for roughly 20% of global dementia costs, while direct social sector costs and informal care costs each account for roughly 40%. The relative contribution of informal care is greatest in the African regions and lowest in North America, Western Europe and some South American regions, while the reverse is true for social sector costs.*

Whatever the real up-to-date costs, we must take action to reduce the burden on individuals and nations. If we do not invest in independent research to develop an effective urine or blood test, cure, and vaccine for each dementia type, the costs will smother economies throughout the world. The costs will cripple developing countries and destabilize the wealthiest.

We have no choice but to invest more in dementia research. No matter which country you live, your economy, security, and the health of your nation rides on us finding a cure or vaccine.

As a scientist, I find it disturbing climate change and independent dementia research are not major priorities. Most governments, businesses, and individuals who can afford to fund dementia remain MIA in the war against dementia.

Before we conclude this section, let's examine the dementia statistics side-by-side in the table below.

DEMENTIA STATISTICS

This table focuses on the number of people with dementia and the number of deaths per 100,000 among the nations chosen for comparison.

NATION	# OF PEOPLE WITH DEMENTIA	DEMENTIA DEATHS PER 100,000 PEOPLE	TOTAL COSTS (US DOLLARS)
Australia	447,115	29.61	$15 billion
Brazil	1 million +	10.71	$16.45 billion
Canadian	747,000	37.30	$10.4 billion
China	16.93 million	19.87	$69 billion
France	1.2 million	30.84	$37.91 billion
Germany	1.5 million	16.99	$57.57 billion
India	4 million	14.57	$28.38 billion
Italy	1.4 million	19.81	$29.96 billion
Japan	4.6 million	7.22	$14.8 billion
Mexico	800,000	3.62	Not available
Spain	800.000+	29.23	$19.98 million
Netherlands	280,000	39.37	$4.44 million
United States	5.8 million	44.41	$290 billion
United Kingdom	850,000	49.18	$26.3 billion

Sources: World Health Rankings[26], Alzheimer's Europe[27], NATSIM[28], Alzheimer's Society[29], Brain Test[30]

Other sources cited in the chapter.

The table comes from my book <u>2020 Dementia Overview</u>, which covers cost and prevalence among comparative nations in greater detail.

Let's next discuss the dementia costs for caregivers.

What Does Dementia Cost Volunteer Caregivers?

Although 41% make less than $50,000, American voluntary caregivers devote a minimum of 18.4 billion hours per year to dementia patients.

Worth $232 billion per year, we underrate the voluntary caregiving heroes in our fight against dementia. This total does not include lost wages for the voluntary caregiver.

According to the Northwestern Mutual C.A.R.E. Study, 67% of voluntary caregivers must cut their living to help pay for the patient's medical care, and 57% end up experiencing financial problems[31].

Adding to the costs of voluntary caregivers, they often end up sick themselves. Caring for loved ones with dementia bankrupts many.

In the early stages, the loved one can still perform most of their daily tasks but will require 24/7 care once the symptoms advance.

Imagine putting your life on hold for years to care, bathe, feed, protect, and take such a heavy load on your shoulders.

Millions of dementia families face the dilemma where the husband and wife both must work in most families to get by. You work as a couple to build stability in your own family, and then, boom, doctors diagnose one of you with dementia.

What Does Dementia Cost Dementia Patients?

When we say patient, past a certain stage in the disease, we refer to family or loved ones. A person who cannot perform daily tasks cannot manage finances, even if they have any left.

Too often, the costs drive entire families into bankruptcy because of dementia costs for a member.

Authorities estimate the average cost per dementia patient is $341,840, with families expected to cover 70 percent.

The costs devastate the average family in the industrial nations.

How are they supposed to afford it in developing countries where the average citizen makes less than one-thousand American dollars per year?

Dementia Recap

Although your dementia research has just begun, you now have a decent overview of Dementia.

In Chapter One, we explored dementia. We turned to several top dementia or medical organizations and compared their definitions.

Chapter two explained Alzheimer's is to dementia what China is to Asia. We listed the 19 dementias. They include:

1. _Dementia with Lewy Bodies_
2. _Parkinson's Disease Dementia_
3. Corticobasal Syndrome
4. Typical Alzheimer's Disease
5. _Posterior Cortical Atrophy_
6. _Down Syndrome with Alzheimer's_
7. _Limbic-predominant Age-related TDP-43 Encephalopathy (LATE)_
8. Early-onset Alzheimer's
9. _Behavioral Variant Frontotemporal Dementia_
10. Progressive Supranuclear Palsy
11. _Nonfluent Primary Progressive Aphasia_
12. Logopenic Progressive Aphasia
13. _Cortical Vascular Dementia_
14. _Binswanger Disease_
15. _Normal Pressure Hydrocephalus_
16. _Huntington's Disease_
17. _Korsakoff Syndrome_
18. _Creutzfeldt-Jakob Disease_
19. Amyotrophic Lateral Sclerosis

Although most the dementia types share similar symptoms, enough to cause misdiagnosis, each has its unique pathology and symptoms.

In chapter three, we explored dementia prevalence in the United States, the UK, and worldwide.

Chapter four examined who is most likely to get dementia. We found Native Americans (those who greeted the first Europeans), and black citizens in the United States and the UK are more likely to get dementia than their white or Asian counterparts.

We also explored the women to men ratio. Women represent two-thirds of Alzheimer's and over sixty percent of dementia cases. We pointed out the Alzheimer's figure skews the dementia numbers because men are more likely to get a minimum of 11 of the 19 primary dementia types.

Chapter four explored the US, UK, global, patient, family, and voluntary caregivers' dementia costs. The staggering numbers are almost as frightening as the medical disorder itself.

We borrowed the following table from *2020 Dementia Overview.*

Dementia Costs & Prevalence

NATION	# OF PEOPLE WITH DEMENTIA	DEMENTIA DEATHS PER 100,000 PEOPLE	TOTAL COSTS (US DOLLARS)
Australia	447,115	29.61	$15 billion
Brazil	1 million +	10.71	$16.45 billion
Canadian	747,000	37.30	$10.4 billion
China	16.93 million	19.87	$69 billion
France	1.2 million	30.84	$37.91 billion
Germany	1.5 million	16.99	$57.57 billion
India	4 million	14.57	$28.38 billion
Italy	1.4 million	19.81	$29.96 billion
Japan	4.6 million	7.22	$14.8 billion
Mexico	800,000	3.62	Not available
Spain	800.000+	29.23	$19.98 million
Netherlands	280,000	39.37	$4.44 million
United States	5.8 million	44.41	$290 billion
United Kingdom	850,000	49.18	$26.3 billion

Sources: World Health Rankings[32], Alzheimer's Europe[33], NATSIM[34], Alzheimer's Society[35], Brain Test[36]

The table comes from 2020 Dementia Overview, which covers cost and prevalence among comparative nations in greater detail.

After reviewing the conservative numbers, and factoring in an aging population, we concluded we must find a cure before it bankrupts millions of families and cripples nations.

Having explained the series and introduced dementia, let's discuss the 19 primary dementia types.

Chapter 5: 19 PRIMARY DEMENTIA TYPES

Why is it important to learn about the most prevalent dementias?

There are several reasons. One, the dementias share similar symptoms and—with no accurate testing—doctors often misdiagnose for one of a hundred or more other possibilities. Two, if a person gets one dementia, more often than not, they develop an overlapping second dementia type, known as mixed dementia. In some cases, three dementia types might develop in later stages.

The pathology, related-proteins, atrophy location, and the resulting symptoms determine dementia classifications.

The more we learn about dementia, dementia types, and subtypes grow.

We once thought of Alzheimer's disease as one sweeping neurological disorder, but now know there is typical Alzheimer's, behavior variant Alzheimer's, posterior cortical atrophy, Early-onset Alzheimer's, and the newest dementia category, LATE, previously misdiagnosed for typical Alzheimer's. If that is not complicated enough, there are 20-40 typical Alzheimer's types.

Depending on the pathology, the three primary progressive aphasia subtypes are either Alzheimer's or frontotemporal-related.

We know there is not one vascular dementia, but three: post-stroke dementia, multi-infarct dementia, and Binswanger disease.

There are two Lewy body dementias; Parkinson's disease dementia and dementia with Lewy bodies. There are also other Parkinson-related neurological disorders.

The series covers the 19 most prevalent dementia types. As noted, several are subtypes, but this work extends each equal status and inquiry

Besides breaking down the twenty most prevalent dementia types, we also discuss subtypes for each.

To reduce repetition, we divide the 19 dementias into the following sections.

Lewy Body/Parkinsonism Related Dementias

1. *Dementia with Lewy Bodies*
2. *Parkinson's Disease Dementia*
3. Corticobasal Syndrome

Alzheimer's Related Dementias

4. Typical Alzheimer's Disease
5. *Posterior Cortical Atrophy*
6. *Down Syndrome with Alzheimer's*
7. *Limbic-predominant Age-related TDP-43 Encephalopathy (LATE)*
8. Early-onset Alzheimer's

Frontotemporal Lobar Degeneration Related Dementias

9. *Behavioral Variant Frontotemporal Dementia*
10. Progressive Supranuclear Palsy

Primary Progressive Aphasia Related Dementias

11. *Nonfluent Primary Progressive Aphasia (nfvPPA)*
12. Logopenic Progressive Aphasia (LPA)

Vascular Dementia

13. *Cortical Vascular Dementia*
14. *Binswanger Disease*

Other Dementias

15. *Normal Pressure Hydrocephalus*
16. *Huntington's Disease*
17. *Korsakoff Syndrome*
18. *Creutzfeldt-Jakob Disease*
19. Amyotrophic Lateral Sclerosis

II. POSTERIOR CORTICAL ATROPHY

Let's shift the focus to the book's topic, posterior cortical atrophy.

Chapter 6: POSTERIOR CORTICAL ATROPHY

Also called Benson's disease, posterior cortical atrophy is an Alzheimer's variant. Although once lumped in with typical Alzheimer's, posterior cortical atrophy diverges in how it attacks the brain.

According to NIH, posterior cortical atrophy "is a neurodegenerative syndrome that is characterized by a progressive decline in visuospatial, visuoperceptual, literacy, and praxic skills. The progressive neurodegeneration affecting parietal, occipital and occipito-temporal cortices which underlies PCA is attributable to Alzheimer's disease (AD) in the majority of patients[37]."

Clinical imaging may or may not show atrophy for posterior cortical atrophy patients, complicating studies, and diagnosis.

The UCSF Weil Institute for Neurosciences Memory and Aging Center defines posterior cortical atrophy.

Posterior cortical atrophy (PCA), also called Benson's syndrome, is a rare, visual variant of Alzheimer's disease. It affects areas in the back of the brain responsible for spatial perception, complex visual processing, spelling, and calculation[38].

While rare compared to typical Alzheimer's, posterior cortical atrophy is more prevalent than several among the twenty most prevalent dementias.

How Prevalent Is Posterior Cortical Atrophy?

PCA accounts for up to 5% of Alzheimer's cases, totaling over 200,000 per year, making it a significant dementia category.

What distinguishes posterior cortical atrophy from regular Alzheimer's?

Whereas Alzheimer's attacks short-term memory, early posterior cortical atrophy symptoms are vision-related.

Posterior Cortical Atrophy Causes

Alzheimer's causes most cases, but Lewy body dementia, Creutzfeldt-Jakob disease, and other neurological disorders also cause posterior cortical atrophy. People develop posterior cortical atrophy when the back of the brain shrinks, damaging the part responsible for visual processing and spatial perception[39].

Diagnosis

To make the correct diagnosis, neurologists and other medical professionals must know vital signs and symptoms, which help establish cause and improve the chances they order the right tests and make the correct diagnosis.

Life Expectancy

With no cure, posterior cortical atrophy life expectancy is 8-12 years from diagnosis[40].

Strikes Younger Than Typical Alzheimer's

Posterior cortical atrophy distinguishes itself from Alzheimer's by striking people when they are younger. PCA symptoms manifest earlier than regular Alzheimer's. Whereas most people do not develop regular Alzheimer's until age 65 or older, posterior cortical atrophy symptoms often manifest when people are in their fifties[41].

Posterior cortical atrophy strikes people younger because of specific damage to the back of the brain. While symptoms might appear to be physical, the damage to the brain causes physical problems.

What Causes Posterior Cortical Atrophy?

While Alzheimer's is the most prominent path to posterior cortical atrophy, Lewy body dementia, or Creutzfeldt-Jakob disease causes a minority of cases.

III. POSTERIOR CORTICAL ATROPHY SYMPTOMS

This section covers symptoms for:

1. Typical Alzheimer's
2. Posterior cortical atrophy
3. Early-onset Alzheimer's
4. LATE
5. Down syndrome with Alzheimer's

The symptoms overlap with these five dementias, so we list the specific symptoms for each type, then compare the likes and differences in the section recap.

Chapter 7: POSTERIOR CORTICAL ATROPHY SYMPTOMS

In this chapter, we cover posterior cortical atrophy symptoms, then show how they manifest through stages.

Posterior cortical atrophy distinguishes itself from Alzheimer's by striking people when they are younger. The contrast makes some ask: *How can Alzheimer's cause posterior cortical atrophy, but the latter's symptoms manifest quicker?*

Excellent question!

The answer lies in how long it takes somebody's Alzheimer's symptoms to show. Although Alzheimer's does not strike people younger than 65, the damage to the brain takes place for decades.

Posterior cortical atrophy strikes people younger because of specific damage to the back of the brain. While symptoms might appear to be physical, the damage to the brain causes physical problems.

A trillion neurons in our brain communicate with each other and different parts of our body. Our bodies do what our brain instructs. We do not move our fingers, speak, walk, or otherwise move our body without our brain, sending the correct signal.

While Alzheimer's is the most prominent path to posterior cortical atrophy, there are other neurological causes such as Lewy body dementia or Creutzfeldt-Jakob disease.

Posterior Cortical Atrophy Symptoms

Posterior cortical atrophy symptoms manifest earlier than regular Alzheimer's. Whereas most people do not develop regular Alzheimer's until age 65 or older, posterior cortical atrophy symptoms often manifest when people are in their fifties[42].

Although posterior cortical atrophy patients maintain writing and nonvisual language skills, they suffer other language and visual impairment.

The following are posterior cortical atrophy symptoms:

- Blurred vision
- Bright light & shiny surface sensitivity
- Coordinated movement impairment
- Depth perception difficulties
- Deteriorating calculation skills
- Double-vision
- Getting lost in familiar places
- Hallucinations
- Inability to see in low light
- Inability to recognize familiar people and objects
- Reading difficulties (trouble following lines of text)
- Trouble pointing and reaching for objects
- Writing impairment

Scientists from the United States, the United Kingdom, Canada, Germany, the Netherlands, Belgium, Italy, France, Brazil, and Spain formed a workshop and established a consensus posterior cortical atrophy classification. They determined space perception and simultanagnosia are frequent symptoms. According to the workgroup, common symptoms include[43]:

- Object perception deficit

55

- Constructional dyspraxia
- Environmental agnosia
- Oculomotor apraxia
- Dressing apraxia
- Optic ataxia
- Alexia Left/right disorientation
- Anterograde memory deficit
- Acalculia Limb apraxia
- Prosopagnosia Agraphia
- Visual field defect
- Disoriented to time and place
- Impaired insight
- Verbal fluency agnosia
- Finger agnosia

We discuss posterior cortical atrophy (PCA) symptoms in the stages section.

IV. POSTERIOR CORTICAL ATROPHY STAGES

In this section, we focus on how posterior cortical atrophy stages progress.

Chapter 8: POSTERIOR CORTICAL ATROPHY STAGES

There are seven stages to Alzheimer's, which we adapt for posterior cortical atrophy. Each stage grows more severe until death in stage seven.

Posterior Cortical Atrophy Stages

Let's summarize the seven posterior cortical atrophy stages, then examine each.

Stage One

During this stage, the disease is brewing, but no symptoms manifest. If a person in stage one goes to the doctor, they could not diagnose the problem.

Stage Two

In stage two, mild symptoms develop. Mild symptoms develop during stage two but make no sense. While looking back, patients and loved ones connect the symptoms but not at the time.

Stage Three

Stage three is the reality stage. While the person and loved ones might not connect the symptoms to the disease, they can no longer dismiss the symptoms as anything but serious.

The mild symptoms should become severe enough to see the doctor during stage three. Doctors diagnose some posterior cortical atrophy cases, but pinpointing the disease remains tricky.

Stage Four

The symptoms grow severe enough during stage four, where posterior cortical atrophy patients require some daily help. If not diagnosed during stage three, doctors should diagnose dementia during stage four.

Stage Five

Known as the moderate or mid-stage, stage five brings brutal deterioration. Posterior cortical atrophy patients experience greater difficulty maintaining any resemblance of a normal life. They are fighting for their survival, identity, life by this point.

The volunteer caregiver's job grows more demanding during this stage.

Stage Six

As devastating as the initial symptoms, diagnosis, and stage five, when the symptoms grow more pronounced, stage six brutalizes the victim and loved ones.

Stage Seven

Posterior cortical atrophy and Alzheimer's symptoms are much the same by stage seven, as patients demand 24/7 care and struggle to think, remember, recognize, articulate, mobilize, or function during this period without substantial help.

Stage seven ends in death, although medical authorities might not list posterior cortical atrophy as the primary cause of death.

Let's now analyze each stage.

Posterior Cortical Atrophy Stage One

In stage one, people are oblivious. The average person is winding down their career, perhaps enjoying grandchildren, and looking forward or dreading retirement.

Stage one is the quiet before the big storm. The patient, their family, colleagues, and friends remain oblivious.

Whatever their normal circumstances, everything will soon change.

Posterior Cortical Atrophy Stage Two

Patients develop mild symptoms during this period that include:

- Arithmetic decline
- Color issues in vision
- Difficulty choosing the correct words
- Difficulty judging distances
- Driving decline (in part because of the inability to judge distances)
- Reading deterioration (trouble following the reading lines)
- Trouble remembering and writing numbers such as phone numbers
- Typing decline
- Vertigo
- Visual decline
- Word selection problems
- Writing problems

Some patients might not develop some listed symptoms until later stages or avoid altogether, but will experience some mild combination of symptoms in stage one.

People often see eye doctors during this period, attributing visual symptoms to age-related vision problems. In most cases, the eye tests show no ophthalmological problems.

Posterior Cortical Atrophy Stage Three

Although symptoms remain mild, they become more difficult to hide or excuse. The number of symptoms accumulates and clear enough to alarm loved ones and associates. Driving becomes impossible in stage three.

Stage three symptoms include:

- Cannot tell time
- Cold sensation and other sensory changes
- Clumsier than usual (can't see well)
- Difficulty negotiating stairs
- Difficulty with eating mechanics
- Dressing problems
- Failure to see objects and people right in front of them
- Forget recent events
- Loses one's place on page while reading
- Spatial judgment decline
- Struggles to learn new tasks
- Struggles to write or process numbers
- Trouble finding items in a handbag, drawers, cabinets, etc.
- Trouble reaching for or pointing to objects
- Word selection difficulty

While a person is unlikely to experience all the listed symptoms, and the symptoms remain mild, stage three symptoms cause tremendous anxiety in many patients. The anxiousness worsens the same symptoms creating it.

Posterior cortical atrophy turned their life upside down.

If the patient gets to the right doctor, and they order the correct tests and make the right referrals, neurologists should diagnose posterior cortical atrophy during stage three.

Posterior Cortical Atrophy Stage Four

Previous symptoms grow worse, and new symptoms develop in stage four. A person grows more dependent each day.

One's ability to cook, dress, bathe, operate basic appliances, and perform daily tasks deteriorates during stage four.

Driving is a thing of the past, and the person now fights to maintain any aspects of normal life. While the brain works, posterior cortical atrophy patients struggle in stage four to execute basic tasks because of visual deterioration.

Other stage-four symptoms include:

- Cannot distinguish between a dollar and a hundred-dollar bill
- Can no longer read
- Failure to tell time
- Inability to stand up, sit down, or walk (might do one or two but not all three)
- Incapable of reading medication labels
- Cannot see some objects right in front of them
- Sees moving easier than static objects
- Trouble navigating familiar and unfamiliar surroundings

A person loses the ability to perform former activities, as symptoms make it difficult to get from room-to-room in one's house.

Many posterior cortical atrophy patients enjoy watching television, in part because it does not force them to do anything but sit still. Unable to read and perform many other activities, many enjoy watching television.

The visual issues deteriorate during this state, where they can no longer recognize loved ones except through voice recognition.

Socializing becomes limited, because of word recognition struggles. Besides speech problems, they either eat with hands or need help feeding during stage four.

Visual and speech problems reduce socializing to memories.

Posterior Cortical Atrophy Stage Five

Visual problems worsen in stage five, and a person requires help with all or most daily activities, including dressing, going to the bathroom, bathing, eating, walking, and most simple tasks.

The world becomes a blur as vision only allows a partial view.

Like the story of the blind men each touching a part of the elephant and describing one part as if it is the whole elephant, somebody suffering posterior cortical atrophy cannot make out an entire object. Frustration and anxiety grow more pronounced.

Other stage five symptoms include:

- Episodic memory declines
- Jerky hands, arms, and other body parts
- Lost sense of body (not knowing one is standing, sitting, or laying
- Most become legally blind during stage five
- Hypersensitivity to light, pain, cold, and other body sensations
- Requires walking assistance because of vision and spatial deterioration
- Trouble or inability to turn around, step forward, and following spatial commands.
- Unexplained headaches
- Word selection difficulty worsen

Stage five posterior cortical atrophy makes people sensitive to sounds. They also feel unbalanced when standing or walking.

One does not plan at this stage, but battles through every event in each day. Patients are not clueless about what is going on around them, but spatial and vision limitations make it impossible to grasp the entirety of any environment.

Life is a struggle, and the only thing easing the discomfort is the love and help of caregivers and loved ones. The patient is far past the point of living on their own.

Posterior Cortical Atrophy Stage Six

People develop different combinations of symptoms listed in stages one through five.

Those blind from non-posterior cortical atrophy causes develop their other senses to compensate for the visual disadvantage. Posterior cortical atrophy patients lack such developmental compensation. While therapists help, posterior cortical atrophy strikes and strips away visual ability through a steady attack.

Posterior cortical atrophy also attacks in other ways described in previous stages, preventing a person from developing other sensual abilities to help overcome vision problems.

The jerking movements in fingers and other body parts are like Parkinson's disease dementia patients experience. Stage six related language problems resemble that experienced by primary progressive aphasia patients. New behavioral issues might resemble behavioral variant frontotemporal dementia (bvFTD).

By stage six, posterior cortical atrophy shares more regular Alzheimer's symptoms, but remains distinctive.

Stage six symptoms include:

- Becomes obsessive
- Behavioral and personality changes
- Cannot recall recent events
- Communication breakdown (trouble comprehending and communicating)
- Delusions (might accuse caregiver of stealing things or being an impostor)
- Develops compulsions
- Further sensory deterioration (might lose the sense of touch)
- Further word collection decline

- Halting speech
- Legally blind
- Lost visual stimulation
- Sitting stooped over
- Sleep disturbances (sleeping during the day like Alzheimer's patients)
- Trouble controlling over-active bowels and bladder
- Withdraws from the surrounding world

Stage six is a horrendous struggle. Unable to live, or perhaps even comprehend, the previous world, severe symptoms limit the ability to experience normal moments, for normal days disappeared long ago.

Posterior Cortical Atrophy Stage Seven

Stage seven is the final chapter in what I hope has been a marvelous and blessed life. We all reach this chapter in our own lives. All humans share a few things, including we are born, live, and die.

By stage seven, patients have long required 24/7 care. Unable to see, walk, dress, eat, use the toilet, or do much of anything without help, one becomes as dependent as a newborn baby.

Many are in some medical facility by now. PCA patients who remain home demand continuous care. If one person has been doing the primary volunteer caregiving, they too are wearing down by this stage and often get sick.

Families and loved ones should step up together by this point and relieve the burden on any one person.

Distinguishing between posterior cortical atrophy and Alzheimer's in stage seven is almost impossible, for both are drifting away.

Unable to recognize loved ones or understand their surroundings, the brain, body, and organs malfunction.

Difficulty swallowing makes eating almost impossible, and maintaining nutrients becomes challenging.

Muscles become rigid, and movement limited.

The cause of death on the birth certificate often says pneumonia or some organ failure, and authorities often list posterior cortical atrophy as the underlying cause.

Posterior Cortical Atrophy Stages Recap

Let's review posterior cortical atrophy symptoms.

Stage One

No symptoms.

Stage Two

In hindsight, patient and loved ones connect the symptoms but fail to connect the dots in real-time.

Stage Three

Mild symptoms become severe enough to see the doctor during stage three. Doctors diagnose some posterior cortical atrophy cases, but pinpointing the disease remains elusive in most cases.

Stage Four

The symptoms grow severe enough during stage four to require some daily assistance. If not diagnosed during stage three, doctors should now diagnose dementia.

Stage Five

Stage five brings brutal deterioration. Posterior cortical atrophy patients experience greater difficulty maintaining any resemblance of a normal life.

Stage Six

This stage brutalizes the victim and loved ones. While not as bad as stage seven, stage six shatters any hopes of fighting off this terrible disease.

Stage Seven

Posterior cortical atrophy and Alzheimer's symptoms are indistinguishable by stage seven. Patients require 24/7 care and struggle to think, remember, recognize, articulate, mobilize, or function during this period.

Patients die in stage seven after a long, devastating battle. The cause of death is often pneumonia.

Like Alzheimer's, posterior cortical atrophy, life expectancy is 8-12 years from diagnosis to death.

Symptoms/Stages Sources: Global Deterioration Scale for Assessment of Primary Degenerative Dementia[44], Alzheimer's Association[45], New York University School of Medicine[46], International Scientific Posterior Cortical Atrophy Criteria Workgroup[47]

V. ALZHEIMER'S RELATED RISK FACTORS

This section covers the Alzheimer's-related dementias' risk factors.

As with symptoms and stages, we devote a chapter each to posterior cortical atrophy and LATE, and then a larger chapter covering typical Alzheimer's disease (AD), early-onset Alzheimer's disease (EOAD), and Down syndrome with Alzheimer's disease (DSAD) because they represent three AD manifestation examples and share risk factors.

Chapter 9: POSTERIOR CORTICAL ATROPHY RISK FACTORS

I often complain we need more independent dementia research. Science cannot say for certain what causes posterior cortical atrophy, nor what risk factors increase one's risks.

While we know Alzheimer's, Lewy body dementia, Creutzfeldt-Jacob disease, and other neurological disorders trigger posterior cortical atrophy, but why?

Does posterior cortical atrophy share Alzheimer's risk factors? While many dementias share some risk factors, we cannot yet ascertain posterior cortical atrophy's risk factors.

I cannot overestimate the government's failure to fund independent medical research for posterior cortical atrophy and other dementias. Their neglect means profiteers fund, and their goals conflict with what doctors and patients need. Because governments and 25 percent of the population controlling ninety percent of the wealth refuse to invest, dementia research remains a slow and tedious process.

Researchers continue to make great progress, but society must invest in independent medical research like it does sports and entertainment if we are to discover exact posterior cortical atrophy causes and risk factors. We also need quick, cheap tests to diagnose each dementia type, vaccines to prevent dementias, and specific medication to treat and cure each dementia type in the early stages.

Those who read several of my books this is a recurring theme. Legitimate medical research progress excites, but under-funded or bias research upsets me.

I remain apolitical in my medical books and research, and independent otherwise, and avoid politics altogether when possible. When I reach a section in my writing on risk factors, however, and science cannot determine exact cause and risk factors, I fume.

I know what citizens spend on self-indulgence and how money governments waste, but yet there is never enough money for medical research.

Please join me in letting your political leaders know this is unacceptable. Ask the politicians to waste less tax money and instead approve funding for posterior cortical atrophy and independent medical research.

Once again, I apologize for the lack of information on risk factors for such a significant neurological disorder. I update my books at least once per year and expect an update to include specific posterior cortical atrophy risk factors.

Until then, we will discuss Alzheimer's risk factors and prevention since posterior cortical atrophy evolves into Alzheimer's disease.

Alzheimer's Disease Risk Factors

Again, I stress science confirms these risk factors for typical Alzheimer's disease (AD) and might not end up identical once researchers advance our knowledge of posterior cortical atrophy.

While science does not know the exact cause (s) of Alzheimer's, dozens of studies confirm several Alzheimer's risk factors. Such knowledge points us towards the habits and, sometimes, medicine to avoid or slow Alzheimer's.

While we might discuss overlapping subjects, this short guide's purpose is to provide a simple course on factors within and beyond our control that increases our chances of getting Alzheimer's.

There is another book in the series that focuses on how to prevent or slow Alzheimer's disease. While the books would seem opposites and are, this book is more a prelude to *How to Prevent or Slow Alzheimer's Dementia*. Science might never have figured out steps we can each take to reduce our chances of Alzheimer's, if not for the decades of studies and research that uncovered the risk factors.

While researchers cannot yet find the cause, they have uncovered several risk factors.

There are two risk factors we have no control: Age and genetics (including Down syndrome).

We will examine sixteen total risk factors

1. Age is the obvious risk factor in Alzheimer's dementia.

2. Alcohol Abuse shares similar symptoms and worsens illnesses that elevate one's risk of getting Alzheimer's.

3. Depression is a symptom and a risk factor in Alzheimer's.

4. Diet can protect or destroy our ability to fight diseases such as Alzheimer's as we age.

5. Down Syndrome is a difficult disease that also carries a fifty percent chance of getting Alzheimer's.

6. Genetics blesses and curses us, and one of the cruelest genes point to early-onset Alzheimer's.

7. High Blood Pressure & Hypertension increases one's risk to brain and heart, and Alzheimer's risk.

8. Inactive Minds are a wasteful danger.

9. Low Body Mass does not feed the brain and body and increases one's risk of Alzheimer's.

10. Low Formal Education increases the risk of Alzheimer's unless one educates themselves or otherwise gains an education as an adult.

11. Obesity increases the chances of many devastating diseases, including Alzheimer's.

12. Physical Inactivity, overweight or not, inflates one's chance of heart and brain disease, including Alzheimer's.

13. Prescription Drugs are double-edged swords. While the right medicine can be a lifesaver, the wrong can be

fatal.

14. Sleep Disorders increase the risk of Alzheimer's.

15. Stress boosts the probability of getting Alzheimer's.

16. Tobacco use is a suicidal march, and one of the catastrophic endings is Alzheimer's disease.

17. Type-2 Diabetes is another suicide march toward Alzheimer's.

Age

The older we get, the more at risk we are for Alzheimer's and all adult diseases. Aging itself, however, does not lead to Alzheimer's or memory loss[48].

Since Alzheimer's (not early-onset) strikes those 65 and older, the older one gets, the greater the risk.

A Department of Molecular Neuroscience, Institute of Neurology, University College London concluded: "The greatest risk factor for Alzheimer's disease is advanced age[49]."

None of us can stop the clock, but too many of us complicate the aging process through bad habits.

Everything else we discuss, from factors beyond our control, such as genetics to habits within our control such as diet, affects how we age. Years of neglect, our mind, and bodies carry consequences as we age. Rather than wait until we get older and have problems, we should establish the eating, sleeping, exercising, and positive habits to ward off the preventable dementias and illnesses.

The healthier we eat, the more we exercise, avoid drugs and alcohol, and develop other healthy habits, the less painful and problematic aging must be for each of us. We achieve good health through sacrifice, smart decisions, and work.

In contrast, eating the wrong foods, weak or nonexistent exercise habits, alcohol or drug abuse, and other bad habits catches up with us and makes aging much more complicated than it must be.

For reasons stated, we list age as a related-risk factor for every disease we examine. It is a repetition worth stressing, for even the healthiest and mightiest are mortals.

We'll reiterate the benefits of positive habits and the consequences of bad habits for aging and health.

Alcohol Abuse

When somebody goes to a doctor with Alzheimer's, they will ask if the person drinks alcohol and how much.

Alcohol's relationship to Alzheimer's remains dubious, but alcohol abuse leads to similar cognitive decline symptoms as Alzheimer's. It also can affect blood pressure and diabetes, two known Alzheimer's risk factors.

Alcohol's relationship with tobacco also complicates the effort to determine if alcohol increases one's risk for Alzheimer's.

The Twin Killers

Alcohol and tobacco are the twin killers, for "smokers drink and drinkers smoke[50]."

How many Alcoholics also Smoke Cigarettes?

Between 80 and 95 percent of alcoholics smoke cigarettes, and 70 percent are heavy smokers[51].

Together, alcohol and tobacco synergize, and each inflicts greater harm than they already do by themselves.

There is a chapter on tobacco, but it is important to know the relationship between alcohol and tobacco. Since abusers use alcohol and tobacco, they work together to destroy the mind and body.

How many Americans die each year because of alcohol?

The CDC attributes "88,000 deaths and 2.5 million years of potential life lost[52]," in the United States to alcohol each year.

How many People Worldwide die per year because of Alcohol?

Worldwide, 3.3 million people die from alcohol each year,

5.9 percent of all deaths[53].

Those statistics should provide an incentive not to abuse alcohol. The only smart choices are none and light alcohol consumption. Anything else, including binge drinking, risks major health consequences, including similar symptoms as Alzheimer's.

Science is still unraveling the connection. Researchers work to determine if alcohol abuse causes Alzheimer's.

Does Alcohol Cause Posterior Cortical Atrophy?

We know drinking over the limit of one drink per day (females) and two drinks per day (males) increases your odds of getting Alzheimer's and dementia. The more you drink, the higher your risk[54].

According to Alzheimer's Society, drinking over the recommended maximum, even sporadic, "increases a person's risk of developing common types of dementia such as Alzheimer's disease and posterior cortical atrophy [55]."

If you exceed the recommended maximum (one drink for a woman, two for a man) and can't cut back on your own, get help. You're on a self-destructive path you need to get off of as fast as possible for your present and future health.

Prevention Measure # 1

Do not drink alcohol or do not drink over one drink over 24 hours.

If you only drink on the weekend but go over the limit, you put yourself at risk for dementia and many other medical problems.

Some studies suggest one drink for women and two for men is acceptable, some even suggesting health benefits. Other studies label even minimum alcohol consumption unsafe.

All studies confirm any amount over two drinks over any 24 hours is dangerous. Studies also warn binge drinking is almost as dangerous as abusing alcohol every day.

The smart choice: Never drink over one drink over any 24 hours.

The smarter choice: Do not drink alcohol!

Depression

Depression is something everybody suffers to various degrees but, by a 1.7 to 1 ration, women are more likely to suffer the disease[56]. Women's greater prevalence of depression might explain their higher rate of Alzheimer's than men.

The Mayo clinic attributes greater risk of depression to women to what makes them different: Puberty, premenstrual problems, pregnancy, postpartum depression, perimenopause, and menopause, but also point to inequality, working a job and managing the home, sexual and physical abuse[57].

While depression strikes women more often, it does immeasurable damage to both sexes.

Depression is Serious!

Too many suspect depression sufferers exaggerate their symptoms, but others are much worse than suspected. Those with advanced (untreated) depression, suffer more than what most of us experience.

If a loved one becomes depressed, show patience, and do what you can to lift their spirits. If they do not come out of the depression in a reasonable time, or it seems serious, convince them to see a doctor.

Untreated, depression increases our risk of a wide range of serious health issues.

Does Depression cause Alzheimer's?

While researchers debate if depression is the cause or a symptom, they agree it increases one's chances of getting Alzheimer's.

One 28-year study of 10,189 people concluded[58]:

> *Depressive symptoms in the early phase of the study corresponding to midlife, even when chronic/recurring, do not increase the risk for*

82

dementia. Along with our analysis of depressive trajectories over 28 years, these results suggest that depressive symptoms are a prodromal feature of dementia or that the 2 share common causes. The findings do not support the hypothesis that depressive symptoms increase the risk for dementia.

While the debate continues, there remains no definitive evidence Depression causes Alzheimer's.

A Royal College of Psychiatric study released in the *British Journal of Psychiatry* confirms the results of other studies. Meryl A. Butters, Ph.D., Department of Psychiatry, University of Pittsburg School of Medicine, explained their findings. "Late-life depression," said Butters, "is associated with an increased risk for all-cause dementia, posterior cortical atrophy, and Alzheimer's disease[59]."

Butters calls for: "clinical trials to investigate the effect of late-life depression prevention on risk of dementia, in particular, posterior cortical atrophy and Alzheimer's disease."

Since we know risk factors, it makes sense to study if treating them reduces the risk to Alzheimer's. The government and those with the money should spend the money on the clinical trials Butters and others urge.

Part of Alzheimer's solution might be to treat other diseases such as depression better.

Why is it difficult to distinguish between Alzheimer's & Depression?

In the early and middle stages, Alzheimer's and Depression behavior resemble each other. With no accurate Alzheimer's test, chances of early misdiagnosis remain high.

"Alzheimer's and depression have some similar symptoms," the Mayo Clinic explained. "Proper treatment improves {the} quality of life[60]."

A study supported by the National Institute of Mental

Health and the National Institute on Aging confirmed the connection between depression and Alzheimer's and calls for more studies. The researchers explained[61]:

> *The most likely links are the following hypothesized mechanisms: 1) vascular disease; 2) alterations in glucocorticoid steroids and hippocampal atrophy; 3) increased deposition of β-amyloid plaques; 4) inflammatory changes; and 5) deficits of nerve growth factors or neurotrophins.*

Several risk factors, including depression, cause similar brain reactions, symptoms experienced by people carrying Alzheimer's.

Widowed

One late-life form of depression is losing a loved one. Those fortunate enough to find lasting love and both live long lives must face a day when one must live without the other.

Is there anything worse than losing one's soulmate? Of life's many jolts, losing one's life partner is the most difficult for some to overcome, sending them deep into a state of depression, many cannot recover.

When you build your life foundation on a deep partnership with another, losing them is a brutal fate. And, our finite existences means one partner in every meaningful relationship is likely to lose the other at some point.

While many factors are contributing to depression, losing a spouse stands out because often it strikes seniors when they are most vulnerable.

Losing people we love is the worst part of life, and more so for recent widows and widowers.

We need more studies!

Alzheimer's remains mysterious. We don't know if Alzheimer's is Type-3 Diabetes, as some suggest, an outgrowth of Depression, or several important factors.

Scientists from the United States and Europe analyzed several studies on the link between depression and Alzheimer's. "These findings thus underscore the possible relation between the two disorders," they concluded, "and the importance of continued research on the common and disparate factors in the etiology of depression and AD {Alzheimer's disease}[62]."

We reviewed dozens of studies on the link, and everyone emphasized the urgency for new research.

Controlled human studies are also a priority I emphasize throughout our books on Alzheimer's and other dementias.

The human and medical costs of depression and Alzheimer's are too high not to fund the research necessary to cure both. Invest in research now and save money for the government and people over the long run.

We monitor ongoing studies and will update this chapter in our 2020 edition. Please seek treatment for any serious or long term depression.

Prevention Measure #2

Avoid or treat depression. We all get depressed but seek help for severe or prolonged depression.

Living with depression is agony.

Depression also increases our risks for many diseases and links to Alzheimer's and other dementias. We must view severe depression with the same urgency as a broken leg.

Turn to your friends, family, and seek professional help if needed. Like if you had a broken leg, you need help if depression causes you to struggle through each day.

Treat severe depression like the serious medical condition it is. Get help!

In the next section, we examine the diet's relationship to Alzheimer's.

Diet

Nobody likes to discuss our unhealthy diets. We make poor food choices, and we pay the price. If we eat too much, we become congested. If we eat wrong over time, we increase our risk of diseases such as Alzheimer's.

Eating a balanced diet is the best way to remain healthy, but many make horrible food choices. Too much sugar, salt, refined grains, corn syrup. Too little vegetables, fruits, salmon, water,

Whether a meat-eater, vegetarian, or vegan, one can build a tasty, healthy diet. However, too many in each group fail this important task.

We help or hurt ourselves through our food choices. We've already pinpointed diet's importance to the aging process and health.

It's also vital for preventing Alzheimer's. Like the body, if we starve the mind from lack of nutrients, or by poisoning it with the wrong choices, there are consequences, and Alzheimer's and dementia are among the worse.

The Mayo Clinic warns the lack of vegetables and fruit in a diet causes Alzheimer's disease[63].

Processed foods contain dangerous amounts of sweeteners, sodium, preservatives, and harmful chemicals. Food manufacturers remove most of the vitamins, minerals, and nutrients during the processing.

If you eat a poor diet loaded with animal fat and processed foods full of sweeteners and artificial preservatives, you're increasing your chances of Alzheimer's.

Western Diet

Many foods in the Western diet increase Alzheimer's risk. We also know no credible medical researcher ever recommended the Western Diet a medical solution to any symptom or illness.

87

The Western Diet is a curse that spreads obesity, Type-2 diabetes, hypertension, and other heart and brain illnesses. Eating regular portions would be harmful enough without most of us eating 2-4 times more than our recent ancestors.

Let's review foods you should avoid in the name of longevity.

10 Foods You Should Not Eat or Drink

1. Alcohol (if you drink, do not exceed one drink per day)
2. Diacetyl is a flavoring added to butter, cheese, cookies, candy, crackers, flour, milk, mixes, and microwave popcorn
3. Processed cheese
4. Medication that begins with "anti"
5. Nitrates added to processed and cured meats
6. Processed meats (bacon, deli meat, ham, etc.)
7. Processed foods
8. Smoked meats (including smoked turkey, ham, etc.)
9. White foods (bread, cakes, pasta, rice, etc.)
10. White sugar

As you see, most white foods (other than Cauliflower & white vegetables) are bad for us.

White Poisons

The following are white foods to avoid:

- White flour
- White rice
- White sugar.

The Western diet uses these poisons in abundance in thousands of recipes

Let's review these high-risk foods.

Alcohol

Alcohol might be a risk factor for Alzheimer's disease, but we know heavy drinking worsens the disease. We also know excessive drinking leads or worsens several of the proven risk factors for Alzheimer's: High blood pressure, Type—2 diabetes, and other direct contributors to Alzheimer's. And we know most those who abuse alcohol also are heavy smokers.

Stick to the maximum level (one drink per 24 hours), and you should be okay. If drinking is not important to you, do not drink. Remember, binge drinking (only abusing on weekends or special events) damages our body much like those who abuse alcohol daily.

Diacetyl

Food process companies add Diacetyl as a flavoring to butter, cheese, cookies, candy, crackers, flour, milk, mixes, and popcorn

Medication that begins with "anti"

Avoid the over the counter, and prescribed drugs beginning with "anti" or have "nitrates" in the name.

Nitrates

Manufacturers use nitrates to process and cure meat.

Processed cheese

They process most cheese, and most contain Diacetyl. If you eat cheese, choose aged, non-processed options.

Processed foods

Avoid all processed food. Any healthy diet avoids processed food and focuses on whole food.

Processed meats

Avoid processed meats.

- Bacon
- deli meat
- ham
- other processed meats

Smoked meats

Including smoked turkey, ham, etc.

White foods

Avoid foods using white flour or white sugar:

- bread
- cakes
- pasta
- white rice
- any food made with white flour or white sugar

Instead, eat whole foods that do not require labels. If there is a label with ingredients, there is processing.

White sugar

Do not stock or use white sugar at home. Do not consume sugar-filled drinks and food outside the home.

Prevention Measure 3

Most people control what they eat and drink.

If we eat processed food loaded in sugar and salt, unhealthy habits increase our risk for dementia and several other fatal diseases.

If we eat whole grains, vegetables, wild fish, and a balanced wholefood diet, healthy habits improve our chances for health and prosperity.

We recommend balance and whole foods such as the Mediterranean diet. Whether you are vegan, vegetarian, eat meat, or whatever you call the diet, it boils down to one primary principle.

Eat a balanced wholefood diet!

Down Syndrome

Most of the risk factors outlined in this book are correctable by developing better habits, but not Down syndrome. Genetics only explains five percent of Alzheimer's cases, but those born with Down syndrome are one example.

People with Down syndrome have a third copy of chromosome 21 when two are normal. Research confirms multiple genes in chromosome 21 elevates one's risk for Alzheimer's.

According to the National Down Syndrome Society, people, sixty or older with Down syndrome stand a 50 percent chance of getting Alzheimer's [64].

Those living with Down syndrome carry a thirty percent chance of getting early-onset Alzheimer's[65].

Alzheimer's disease affects about 30% of people with Down syndrome in their 50s. By their 60s, this number comes closer to 50%.

Science has made progress

In the eighties, the life expectancy of those with Down syndrome was under 25 years. Advance three decades and science upped the number beyond sixty[66].

What to do if a loved one has Down syndrome?

See your doctor and follow their advice, or see a new doctor if you do not trust the competency or ethics of the first.

Down Syndrome is not an automatic sentence for Alzheimer's

As the National Down Syndrome Society stresses[67]:

While all people with Down syndrome are at

risk, many adults with Down syndrome will not manifest the changes of Alzheimer's disease in their lifetime. Although risk increases with each decade of life, at no point does it come close to reaching 100%.

We also recommend learning and avoiding the foods and habits that cause Alzheimer's and the dementias and instead eat a whole food diet and practice healthier habits.

Down syndrome is an AD risk factor, no fault of the victims. We hope science soon finds a means to prevent Alzheimer's in 100 percent of people with Down syndrome.

Gender

While scientists have discovered nothing to confirm gender plays a direct role in Alzheimer's development, females make up two-thirds of American Alzheimer's victims[68].

Considering women live longer, we might expect them to suffer a higher rate of disease than men.

Studies suggest; however, women suffer a much higher incidence of Alzheimer's than men, even when accounting for them living longer[69].

Jessica L. Podcasy, MS, and C. Neill Epperson, MD led research on Sex and Gender in Health, University of Pennsylvania Department of Psychiatry explain[70]:

> *Advanced age is the strongest predictor; however, sex and gender differences have been noted in prevalence, clinical manifestation, disease course, and prognosis. Data from the Framingham Study, which enrolled a total of 2611 cognitively intact participants (1550 women and 1061 men) and followed up on many for 20 years, indicated that for a 65-year-old man, remaining lifetime risk of AD was 6.3% (95% confidence interval [CI], 3.9 to 8.7) and remaining lifetime risk of developing any dementing illness was 10.9% (95% CI, 8.0 to 13.8); corresponding risks for a 65-year-old woman were 12% (95% CI, 9.2 to 14.8) and 19% (95% CI, 17.2 to 22.5), almost twice that of men.*

Let's review a study at the University of Luxembourg to see how their results compare.

"Men have a 1 in 11 chance of developing the disease," according to the lead scientist Dr. Enroco Glaab, "but yet for women, the odds are 1 in 6 even when accounting for their longer life span[71]."

The Luxembourg results confirm women are almost twice as likely as men to get Alzheimer's.

From childhood anxiety and depression to childbirth to motherhood, life is never easy for women. But, such unique female hardships do not doom women.

What one eats, how much they exercise, and how one avoids certain things under our control can reduce one's chances.

We need studies comparing healthy women to men who eat unhealthy diets, do not exercise, and are overweight.

My guess is these men with unhealthy habits have a higher chance of Alzheimer's than women who live healthier lifestyles. What we know is women and men can reduce our chances of Alzheimer's by eating healthy, working out, engaging and challenging our minds, and otherwise following scientific advice.

What if Men suffered Alzheimer's the same rates as women?

I am a man, but also a humanist and medical researcher. The men who dominate business and government would devote more money towards Alzheimer's and dementia research if the disease struck middle-aged men instead of older women.

The lengths our leaders go to send young Americans to the other side of the world to launch a war we should not fight should get the politicians thrown out of office. So should their reluctance to invest in legitimate medical research, and their lesser interest in research that benefits women in greater numbers offend humanity.

Sorry for the outburst. Beller Health books are for everybody, no matter one's politics, religion, race, gender, or any other division. The research and books for this book series are apolitical. We follow the research and science and hold no hidden agenda. There is no room for partisanship, bias, or anything else that corrupts research. Our goal is to promote and defend impartial scientific research and to analyze and report the findings.

Can everybody agree our politicians and leaders hold misplaced priorities? When I call them out, it is not a partisan attack, for I could not care less about which party they come. When engaged in this book, my colleagues and I place victims, cures, knowledge, symptoms, risks over political party or group identification.

Here, as a male medical researcher, it is clear women do not always receive equal medical attention as men, and the gap grows more pronounced with minority females.

My colleagues and I call for greater funding into Alzheimer's research, and specific studies to identify why women are twice as likely to carry Alzheimer's as men.

Does genetics explain the greater Alzheimer's prevalence in women?

Genetics might play a role, but environmental factors such as women's products uncommon for men also might explain the disparity. It is inconclusive.

Genetics

Genetics causes less than five percent of Alzheimer's cases. [72] Science has found several genes that increase the odds but do not guarantee one gets Alzheimer's. If a parent or sibling has the disease, it increases one's chances of Alzheimer's.

Dozens of large studies over 30 years reviewed[73]:

> *To date, more than 20 non-APOE-related loci exhibit {a} nominally significant association with disease risk in systematic meta-analyses of the available AD genetic literature7. These findings implicate many of the potential culprits that have long been believed to be involved in the development of neurodegeneration and dementia (such as APP metabolism, Ab degradation and clearance, signal transduction, tau dysfunction, protein trafficking, cholinergic deficits, cholesterol metabolism and the homeostasis of heavy metals).*

Genetic Relation to Early-onset Alzheimer's

Genetics plays a large role in early-onset, which accounts for less than ten percent of Alzheimer's.

How many Americans have early-onset Alzheimer's?

Of the 5.5 million Americans with Alzheimer's, over 200,000 have early-onset[74].

How do parents weigh into the equation?

"A child whose biological mother or father carries a genetic mutation for early-onset FAD has a 50/50 chance of inheriting that mutation," reported the National Institute on Aging. "If the mutation is inherited, the child has a very strong probability of developing early-onset FAD[75]."

Each parent or sibling with Alzheimer's increases your chances of getting the disease.

However, Alzheimer's threatens all humans, and we all have the same prevention plan. What we control is establishing good habits and reducing our bad habits that increase our chances of getting Alzheimer's.

Genetic Relation to Late-onset Alzheimer's

From the data collected, genetics is not a high risk for late-onset Alzheimer's. We do not know the specific cause of Alzheimer's, but the National Institute on Aging claims, "having one form of the apolipoprotein E (APOE) gene on chromosome 19—does increase a person's risk[76]."

The next step

The next step is to find a means to stop the risk genes in their tracks. A study released in *Nature Medicine* is one of the more promising because it used human genes, instead of testing on lab rats.

The Gladstone Institutes study lead author Yadong Huang explained the importance. "Drug development for Alzheimer's disease has been largely a disappointment over the past ten years," said Huang. "Many drugs work beautifully in a mouse model, but so far they've all failed in clinical trials. One concern within the field has been how poorly these mouse models mimic human disease[77]."

While animal testing has helped advance medicine, what works on rats might not work on humans. The Gladstone Institutes scientists in the *Nature Medicine* study discovered how apoE4 increases the risk of Alzheimer's. More importantly, the scientists devised a way to convert it into a "harmless apoE3-like version[78]."

While scientists must conduct more studies before we see any such treatment available to the public, such breakthroughs might one day provide a godsend for those who carry the risk genes.

High Blood Pressure And Hypertension

For most people, bad habits lead to high blood pressure and hypertension, raising the risk of heart disease and Alzheimer's. Not to shame anybody, but we humans accumulate bad habits, which have consequences, and one is high blood pressure.

We examine how high blood pressure increases Alzheimer's risks.

How does high blood pressure increase Alzheimer's risks?

Studies suggest high blood pressure inhibits the protein ACE, which breaks down the harmful amyloid protein associated with Alzheimer's.

American Academy of Neurology Study

A study published in the *American Academy of Neurology* followed 1,288 people, 65 percent women, and found Alzheimer's "pathology showed an association of a higher mean SBP with a higher number of tangles[79]."

Funded by the National Institutes of Health, study author Zoe Arvanitakis, MD, MS, of the Rush Alzheimer's Disease Center at Rush University Medical Center in Chicago said reported high systolic blood pressure increases the risk of brain lesions by 46 percent or more.

"When looking for signs of Alzheimer's disease in the brain at autopsy," Arvanitakis said, "researchers found a link between higher average late-life systolic blood pressure across the years before death and a higher number of tangles[80]."

How is blood pressure measured?

We gauge blood pressure by measuring two pressures, systolic (top number) and diastolic (bottom number).

Systolic Pressure

Systolic pressure measures artery and blood vessels pressure per heartbeat.

Diastolic Pressure

Diastolic pressure measures the pressure between heartbeats.

What is normal blood pressure, high blood pressure, and hypertension?

New Blood Pressure Reading Measurements

The American Heart Association established new guidelines for blood pressure readings. Let's review the chart of their updated recommendations:

BP Category	Systolic BP		Diastolic BP
Normal	<120 mmHg	and	<80 mmHg
Elevated	120-129 mmHg	and	<80 mmHg
Hypertension: stage 1	130-139 mmHg	or	80-89 mmHg
Hypertension: stage 2	$\geq$140 mmHg	or	$\geq$90 mmHg
Hypertensive emergency	>180 mmHg	and/or + target organ damage	>120 mmHg

Source: American College of Cardiology/American Heart Association Task Force on Clinical Practice Guidelines[81].

The new guidelines lower the maximum normal, elevated,

and hypertension blood pressure levels.

High Blood Pressure

How many people have high blood pressure?

United States

In another indictment of the modern Western diet and lifestyle, the American Heart Association claims 103 million, almost half of American adults, have high blood pressure or hypertension.

According to Dr. Paul Muntner, co-chair of the American Heart Association report, the updated numbers are but the start of bad news. "With the aging of the population and increased life expectancy," said Muntner, "the prevalence of high blood pressure is expected to continue to increase[82]."

Worldwide

World Health Organization reports high blood pressure causes 7.5 million deaths, 12.8 percent of annual fatalities, and that one billion people live with untreated hypertension[83].

The silent killer

High blood pressure is known as the silent killer because, much like Alzheimer's, it shows no outward symptoms in the earlier stages.

What causes high blood pressure?

Age

Despite our protests, the older we reach, the greater our risks to high blood pressure, heart disease, and Alzheimer's.

Alcohol abuse

If we drink over one drink per 24 hour period, we risk serious consequences, and high blood pressure is one.

Excess salt (sodium)

Most fast and restaurant food has too much salt, as does canned foods. Despite food already too salted, the first thing the average person does when the food arrives is dash or shovel more salt.

Overloading sodium is a deadly habit.

Family history

A family history of blood pressure increases our risks. Genetics might play a role in rare cases, but bad habits cause high blood pressure and pass along within families.

Illegal drugs

Many illegal drugs cause significant health risks. Different drugs attack specific areas of the body and mind. One side effect of certain illegal drug use is high blood pressure.

Other medical conditions

Diabetes, kidney disease, and sleep apnea elevate blood pressure.

Overweight or obesity

Being overweight leads to diabetes and high blood pressure.

Physical inactivity

Related to being overweight is physical inactivity.

Prescribed Medication

I want to be the first to salute modern medicine for the many breakthroughs that extend and improve our lives, but—because of an inadequate health care system—the average doctor writes prescriptions faster than the best illegal drug dealer can unload their product.

Some medication is a godsend, while the other is a demon-send, for the side effects too often offset any potential benefit.

Race

African Americans are much more likely to get high blood pressure than the rest of the population.

Stress

Continuous or critical stress can lead to anxiety and high blood pressure. While minimizing and controlling stress is easier said than done, it might save our lives.

Tobacco

Of the million reasons to avoid tobacco, it increases the risk of high blood pressure.

Too little potassium

Related to high levels of salt (sodium), the Western Diet has too little potassium. Avoiding or combatting high blood pressure require we consume more potassium in our foods than sodium. Instead, most American foods are high in sodium and low in potassium.

Prevention Measure 4

To avoid strokes, vascular disease, and dementia, one must control their blood pressure.

If you have or want to avoid high blood pressure, please include the following eight recommendations:

1. Improve your diet by eating more fruit, vegetables, and whole grains[84].
2. Exercise. Run, walk, swim, hike, whatever you will do several times per week.
3. If you use any tobacco product, stop!
4. Minimize stress. We all experience stress, but we control how we respond.
5. If you are overweight, combine a diet and exercise plan that will help reduce it to an acceptable level.
6. Try to build a three to one ratio of potassium to sodium in your diet.
7. If you drink alcohol, limit it to one drink per 24 hours.
8. If you use illegal drugs, stop.

Inactive Mind

As dangerous as a dormant body is an inactive mind.

Our ancestors traveled by foot and did everything by hand, so they received continuous physical exercise. If they hoped for longevity, their minds focused on finding food and shelter and avoiding hostile animals and humans. Survivors among our ancestors did so because they developed and practiced the physical and mental habits to survive.

Modern humans spend too much time sitting at work, then on the sofa watching television in the evening. The combination of inactivity and poor diets do not provide the brain stimuli needed for growth. Unhealthy diets starve the brain of important nutrients, while not exercising our brain allows it to weaken like any neglected muscle.

Half of Americans have high blood pressure and are overweight, a combination lowering the human physical and cognitive potential. We know how to eat healthier, engage in brain stimuli, and develop our bodies in ways our ancestors could not have fathomed.

Yet half of Americans, and a similar number of global citizens, scoff at the information and tools and instead pursue a life of indulgence, recklessness, and unnecessary danger. We are stubborn!

How is Brain Exercise related to Alzheimer's?

A study released in the *American Academy of Neurology* concluded[85]:

> *How often older people read a newspaper,*
> *play chess, or engage in other mentally*
> *stimulating activities is related to {the} risk of*
> *developing Alzheimer's disease, according to a*
> *new study. The study found a cognitively active*
> *person in old age was 2.6 times less likely to*
> *develop dementia and Alzheimer's disease than a*

cognitively inactive person in old age. This
association remained after controlling for past
cognitive activity, lifetime socioeconomic status,
and current social and physical activity.

A study in the Journal of the American Medical Association analyzed 801 older priests, brothers, and nuns. Robert S. Wilson, Ph.D., and the team found: "frequent participation in cognitively stimulating activities is associated with reduced risk of AD[86]."

Prevention Measure 5

Exercise your brain! Free, challenge, engage, and stimulate your mind! As the *Swiss Medical Weekly* says of cognitive activity, "Use it or lose it[87]."

Among the recommended cognitive activity:

- Keep learning. Learn a new language. Study history. The important thing is to keep learning, which expands the mind
- Play games, thinking games like chess
- Read books
- Write a diary
- Write letters
- Read a credible daily newspaper (or ten or twenty online)
- Attend a social function
- Call (or better visit) family and friends

Challenging the mind is rewarding and fun. History, art, science, nature, and several avenues provide fabulous brain exercise. Pursue things that inspire, move, challenge, and feeds your passion and mind.

Low Formal Education

The lower the level of formal education, the higher one's Alzheimer's risk.

I do not believe formal education is necessary, but education is the key.

Three of the great American presidents were self-taught men. Those three men—Abe Lincoln, Harry Truman, and Dwight Eisenhower—are three of our most revered presidents.

The one thing the three had in common is they read and worked harder to learn than their counterparts who received formal education.

My point is one can always read. If you cannot read, turn to somebody who will teach you and spend the rest of your life reading.

The University of Southern California, Department of Psychology Research

A University of Southern California team analyzed 88 studies and 71 articles to determine if lower education levels increased risks of Alzheimer's. "Lower education was associated with a greater risk for dementia in many but not all studies," reported Margaret Gatz, Ph.D. "Of the 13 studies that analyzed the relationship between low education and risk for AD, seven studies reported significant effects such that lower education was associated with an increased risk for AD."

Study Released in the American Journal of Epidemiology

A study released in the *American Journal of Epidemiology* found a lower a woman's educational level, the higher their risks of Alzheimer's[88].

Study Published in the Medical Journal for the American Academy of Neurology

A study from Finland published in the American Academy of Neurology followed almost 1,400 people for 21 years. They found[89]:

> *People who don't finish high school are at a higher risk of developing dementia and Alzheimer's disease compared to people with more education, regardless of lifestyle choices and characteristics such as income, occupation, physical activity, and smoking,*

University of Cambridge Study

A team of researchers from the UK and Finland examined the brains of 872 who took part in three large aging studies, so their past was well-documented.

"Over the past decade, studies on dementia have consistently showed that the more time you spend in education, the lower your risk of dementia," said co-author Dr. Hannah Keage of the University of Cambridge. "For each additional year of education, there is an 11% decrease in risk of developing dementia."

There appears to be a link to educational level and Alzheimer's, but again I caution not to paint with too broad of a brush. Those with lower education levels also make less money, receive inferior health care, live in homes and neighborhoods that pose greater health risks, and face a different norm than do the middle or upper classes.

I believe education matters, whether it be formal. If a person reads, writes, thinks, engages their mind, avoids trouble, minimizes stress, enjoys life, knows history, embraces science, and practices the Golden Rule, they will overcome their lack of formal education.

Prevention Measure 6

Reversing the risk is not a matter of hanging a fancy diploma on the wall, but about challenging and exercising your mind, the same thing we recommended for the inactive mind risk.

Although enrolling at a community college (or four year school) is a great option, learning is the key.

This world is a great adventure. Study the stars. Learn a new skill. Study the world around you. Keep a journal. Play chess. Read books. Write poetry. Develop art. Learn! Learn! Learn! Every single day of your life!

Obesity

Like the rest of the book, his section is not about shame. By the time we reach forty, most of us are battling body fat and more so with the past couple generations where the average person has eaten more and exercised less.

Type-2 Diabetes is a serious disease that leads to a variety of other, even worse, diseases. Here's the difference between Type-2 Diabetes and the average killer disease; Type-2 Diabetes results from almost 100 percent eating too large of helpings of the wrong food, and engaging in too little physical exercise.

Also related to diet and exercise is obesity, which leads to Type-2 Diabetes, which causes strokes, which leads to Alzheimer's disease[90].

Obesity is the front and center of contemporary health issues. If you want to avoid Alzheimer's and other severe illnesses, it's vital to control your weight.

Study Published in the United States Library of Medicine National Institutes of Health

A group of scientists reviewed longitudinal epidemiological studies to determine obesity and diabetes' risk factors for Alzheimer's. They concluded: "Obesity and diabetes significantly and independently increase risk for AD[91]."

A Second Study Published in the United States Library of Medicine National Institute of Health

The study followed 10,276 women and men for almost ten years to determine the relationship between obesity and Alzheimer's. They concluded: "Obesity in middle age increases the risk of future dementia independently of comorbid conditions[92]."

A Third Study Published in the Journal of the American Medical Association

The Cardiovascular Risk Factors, Aging, and Dementia

Study analyzed studies from 1972 to 1987, then recruited 1,449 people for an average 21 year follow-up examination. They concluded: "Obesity at midlife is associated with an increased risk of dementia and AD later in life[93]."

The evidence appears clear that obesity increases the risks of Alzheimer's (and several other diseases). If you or loved ones are overweight, please take steps to reduce your weight within the excepted weight range for your height and gender.

Weight is something ninety-plus percent of us can defeat with a solid plan and will power. It will not be easy but will be one of your greatest personal accomplishments, and among your proudest.

Physical Inactivity

Related to obesity is physical inactivity. The average American (human) consumes too much food, and the only way to balance the extra calories is to remain active.

The modern world offers an abundance of food for anybody who can afford, and a variety of movies, television series, social media options, and other gadgets that park one in a seat for hours.

If we follow every fad, we all end up with a weight problem, which leads to Type-2 diabetes, which increases the risks for cancer, heart attacks, strokes, Alzheimer's, and other dementias.

Study Released in the Journal of the American Medical Association

A New York study followed 1,880 people without dementia over 15 years. "In this study," said Nikolaos Scarmeas, MD, "both higher Mediterranean-type diet adherence and higher physical activity were independently associated with reduced risk for AD[94]."

Systematic Review of Several Studies

This systematic review found physical inactivity increased cognitive decline risk in 20 of 24 longitudinal studies[95].

A Second Systematic Review of Several Studies

These scientists and researchers analyzed dozens of studies. They concluded[96]:

The majority of longitudinal epidemiological studies have clearly shown associations between physical activities and the risk of cognitive decline in a dose-response manner suggesting

113

*that physical activities may delay the onset of
AD as well as the risk of cognitive decline and
mortality.*

Our bodies break down when we do not engage ourselves
in continuous physical activity. Not getting enough exercise is
as bad for our minds as our bodies.

Prevention Measure 7

Walk. Swim. Run. Hike. These and other physical activities strengthen your body and mind and reduce your chances of Alzheimer's.

Also, lift light weights or perform resistance exercises three days per week.

If you enjoy life, take steps to enhance health and longevity. Be active!

Prescription Drugs

According to Science Daily, "Multiple drug classes commonly prescribed for common medical conditions are capable of influencing the onset and progression of Alzheimer's disease[97]."

A Harvard study warns that benzodiazepines increase the risk of Alzheimer's and poses the greatest risk to older people[98].

We require more tests on the long-range effects of benzodiazepines and other prescription drugs. While we might know the short-term effects of some of these drugs, they conduct too few studies to determine their long-term consequences.

Harvard Medical School reviewed two studies[99]:

> *In two separate large population studies, both benzodiazepines (a category that includes medications for anxiety and sleeping pills) and anticholinergics (a group that encompasses medications for allergies and colds, depression, high blood pressure, and incontinence) were associated with an increased risk of dementia in people who used them for longer than a few months. In both cases, the effect increased with the dose of the drug and the duration of use.*

These drugs are dangerous and in many prescription and over-the-counter drugs. There have not been enough long-term studies for thousands of other drugs to know if they increase Alzheimer's risks (or other serious health risks).

A Review Published in the British Medical Journal

This review focused on 300,000 seniors, their medical use, and the risks of Alzheimer's and other dementias. They found those who took medication containing anticholinergic increased their risk of Alzheimer's and other dementias by a minimum of 11 percent. The number rose to 30 percent for those who consumed the most anticholinergic[100].

Worst Pills

Worst Pills, Best Pills lists 136 drugs that cause cognitive impairment, including drug-induced dementia. Their list includes most of the drugs linked to a greater risk of Alzheimer's, including anticholinergic, benzodiazepines, eszopiclone, opiates, zolpidem (AMBIEN), zaleplon, sedatives, tricyclic antidepressants[101].

If your doctor prescribes any medication, check to see if the drugs contain any of the above. Make certain your doctor knows of the higher risks of Alzheimer's and other dementias and ask if taking the medication is worth the risk.

Also, watch out for any of these ingredients in over-the-counter drugs. Better yet, try to avoid most over-the-counter drugs. Most get credit for illnesses that go away on their own and have dozens of side effects worse than the modest symptoms they claim to cure.

A Broken System

The problem with the average drug dealer, legal or illegal, is they place profit over their fellow human being's welfare.

Big Pharmaceutical

Pharmaceutical is in business (like those in other industries) to make a profit. Anybody who works for a corporation knows corporate (and board members) profits are the priority. For this discussion, the statement is a fact and does not weigh in on the ethics. My point is they are there to profit, not for the public good.

Insurance Companies

Most people have sorry insurance. The average Americans choose from "insurance" options resembling fool's gold. Expensive premiums, high deductibles, and low coverage are bankrupting American families and a drag on the national and global economy.

The Affordable Care Act

A half-baked plan intended to evolve into real insurance, the Affordable Care Act has stagnated in Congress and remains nothing more than catastrophic coverage forced on those who cannot afford it, and does little to help them with health care.

Congress

The political parties must advance the coverage into real insurance like Congress did Social Security.

Democrats must admit the Affordable Care Act does not provide Americans legitimate and affordable insurance, and Republicans need to help improve the Affordable Care Act or offer an alternative proposal (something they did not do in all this time they complained and sabotaged the Affordable Care Act). Everybody in Congress should be ashamed of forcing poor people to buy catastrophic insurance dressed up as medical coverage. The poor cannot afford $10,000 deductibles before any coverage kicks in!

I call on Congress and politicians around the world to take Alzheimer's, dementia, and people's health care serious. Stop playing political soccer and using people's health as your ball.

Lower the costs and improve the coverage for all people!

Doctors

General practitioners today fight to remain in business like everybody else and sorry insurance policies has turned the typical doctor visit into:

- Fill out a lot of paperwork you have already filled out (in the digital age!)
- Camp in the waiting room for up to an hour or more
- A nurse takes you to a room and perhaps takes your blood pressure and asks you a few questions like what are your symptoms

POSTERIOR CORTICAL ATROPHY

- Wait in the room for another fifteen minutes or longer before the doctor arrives
- The doctor spends five minutes with you and writes one or more prescriptions

Doctors write too many prescriptions, and Americans consume too many legal and illegal drugs. If required, medications work right and do not cause a reaction worse than what they are curing, and we endorse such prescriptions 100 percent.

But, the herd them in and out medical system in the United States and most the world does not allow doctors to get to know their patients, learn their full symptoms, or to counsel them on safer, natural options that work as well or better than some of these drugs.

To herd them through like sorry health insurance demands, and to prevent getting sued, doctors write prescriptions only five minutes after seeing a patient. The continuous prescriptions allow doctors to claim they treated symptoms, and moves you along to the pharmacy to fill your prescriptions, as the pharmaceutical companies demand.

The doctor, Big Pharmaceutical, and insurance companies get paid, while the patient too often gets the shaft.

If doctors are okay with getting paid and looking the other way, continue as usual. If you want more than our medical system offers, speak out!

119

Prevention Measure 8

Do yourself a favor and avoid or minimize prescription drugs. But how?

What is a person to do?

Be proactive. Eat right, exercise, avoid stress, and do what we must to achieve ultimate health.

Whether you are one of the fortunate with quality medical insurance and care or one of the many with bad or no coverage, our best option is to feed and exercise our bodies and minds like we deserve. Otherwise, we are cheating ourselves.

If you are sick, listen to your doctor, but ask about a prescription's side effect or if there is a natural alternative treatment that would work as well or better. If you take medication, do not take more than the prescription dictates. Remember, avoiding long term use of any medication is best, so try to take natural steps to get off the medication as soon as possible.

Closing Note

Do not stop taking any medication you are already taking without consulting your doctor. If you have a problem requiring medication and your doctor prescribes it, take as directed.

Minimize it!

Sleep Disorder

We need our sleep, so our body and mind can cleanse and reboot for the next grueling 16 or 17 hours. Humans require 7-8 hours of sleep, and as much deep-sleep as possible.

Many things keep us up at night. Stress. Depression. Guilty conscience. Fears. Jealousies. Spite. We eat the wrong foods, too close to bedtime. Allergies and dozens of other diseases keep us awake when we should be sleeping.

Even if nothing is wrong with us, there are trains, automobiles, airplanes, neighbors, and other modern noises that deprive us of valuable sleep. Our challenge is to overcome the noise pollution and get sleep.

Dr. Ronald Petersen, Alzheimer's Disease Research Center, Mayo Clinic, Rochester, Minnesota, investigated sleep apnea's link to Alzheimer's.

"Not only could long-term sleep deprivation raise your risk for dementia {Alzheimer's}," said Dr. Peterson, "research has shown that, over time, people who don't sleep enough also may be at an increased risk for other health problems, including high blood pressure, heart disease, and diabetes[102]."

Note that high blood pressure, heart disease, and diabetes also increase the risks of Alzheimer's.

Tests suggest sleep apnea increases the risk of Alzheimer's by developing a higher level of beta-amyloid protein than those who sleep well.

Let's review if sleep apnea increases the risk of Alzheimer's.

New York University School of Medicine

A New York University School of Medicine study found that 30 to 80 percent of seniors experience sleep apnea. "Those with sleep apnea accumulated amyloid plaque," explained study spokesperson Dr. Ricardo Osorio, "which could trigger

Alzheimer's in the future[103]."

A Review in Science Direct

A *Science Direct* study probed dozens of studies and concluded: "Clinical studies suggest an increased incidence of Alzheimer's disease in sleep apnea patients[104]."

University of California Study

Another University of California study released in the *Journal of the American Medical Association* focused on older women in their eighties. The study concluded those suffering sleep apneas were twice as likely to develop Alzheimer's or another dementia in the next five years as those who slept uninhibited[105].

The studies are consistent that sleep apnea causes cognitive impairment and increases the chance of Alzheimer's and the dementias.

Prevention Measure 9

Too many people consider sleep optional. Others suffer medical issues that inhibit sleep. Both increases risk for dozens of fatal disorders, including Alzheimer's and several dementias.

We recommend you get one of the watch-like devices and monitor your sleep to measure your total sleep and deep sleep. A person requires seven to eight hours of sleep per night, and as much deep sleep as possible.

If you are not getting enough sleep, you might feel sleepy during the day. Trouble remaining awake during the day is a warning sign, so take it seriously.

A few pointers.

- Establish firm times to go to bed and get up.
- Avoid alcohol
- Do not eat spicy foods.
- Avoid any habits, foods, or activities that keep you up at night.
- Use white noise to minimize noise pollution
- Meditate

You must sleep without sleeping pills, which cause too many side effects. Try the listed recommendations and otherwise search for natural means to enhance your sleep.

Get seven to eight hours sleep; no more, no less.

Stress

Follow Bobby McFerrin's advice: Don't worry, be happy[106]. Stress kills humans and raises your risks to Alzheimer's[107].

Unmanaged stress causes anxiety, attacking your insides for months, years, or even decades. Stress and anxiety cause a high rate of Beta-amyloid plaque.

Why is Beta-amyloid a problem?

Beta-amyloid

Let's turn to Director Christopher Rowe of the nuclear medicine department and Center for PET at Austin Hospital in Melbourne, Victoria, Australia. The Australian team studied Beta-amyloid.

"Beta-amyloid is associated with brain dysfunction - even in apparently normal elderly individuals," said Rowe, "providing further evidence it is likely related to the fundamental cause of Alzheimer's disease[108]."

How do Studies Connect Stress to Alzheimer's?

Let's review a few studies and reviews to determine stress's relationship to Alzheimer's.

Wisconsin School of Medicine Review

One of the interesting presentations at the *Alzheimer's Association International Conference* in London was a Wisconsin School of Medicine test measuring stress's relationship to Alzheimer's. The researchers studied 1,320 people[109]:

> *Every stressful event was equal to 1.5 years of brain aging across all participants, except for African-Americans, where every stressful event was equal to 4 years of brain aging.*

That is horrible news for everybody, and numbers African-Americans should pay particular attention. When people say stress is a killer, they are not joking. We plan a book on the added stress factor for African-Americans, Native-Americans (ones here when the Europeans arrived), other minorities, and poor of every type, including European descendants. Most Americans stress, but those at the bottom must carry an even greater load.

The University of Wisconsin study: "concluded that the participants from the most disadvantaged areas performed worse in every aspect of cognitive testing and had higher levels of biomarkers for Alzheimer's."

Those climbing from the bottom face many stressful obstacles, causing constant and severe stress. All classes of modern humans stress, the consequences often are fatal, so we must learn to reduce stress, avoid it when possible, and otherwise minimize.

Let's turn to some other studies and reviews to determine how stress increases the risks of Alzheimer's.

Review Published in Current Opinion in Psychiatry

The lead author, Dr. Linda Mah, Department of Psychiatry, University of Toronto, and team reviewed several large studies.

"Pathological anxiety and chronic stress are associated with structural degeneration and impaired functioning of the hippocampus and the prefrontal cortex," said Dr. Mah, "which may account for the increased risk of developing neuropsychiatric disorders, including depression and dementia {Alzheimer's}[110]."

Chronic stress is dangerous but leads to a greater threat, anxiety. In the classroom, workplace, traffic, lines at stores, and in the comfort of one's home, minimizing stress should be a top priority. We can blow our top dozens of times per day in the modern rat race.

Don't do it!

Moody, Jealous, Worrisome Women have Higher Alzheimer's Risk

A study published in the American Academy of Neurology followed 800 women for 38 years to determine if stress increased their risk of Alzheimer's. Lead author Lena Johansson, Ph.D., at the University of Gothenburg, spoke for the group of researchers.

"Women who are anxious, jealous, or moody and distressed in middle age," Johansson said, "may be at a higher risk of developing Alzheimer's disease later in life[111]."

Although the study only tested women, other studies suggest men also carry a higher risk of Alzheimer's if they worry too much, are moody, or always jealous about something or someone.

Men and women must reduce the stress in our lives and lessen our risks to Alzheimer's, other dementias, and fatal health issues.

Prevention Measure 10

How important is managing stress?

Let's turn to Harvard Medical School.

Harvard Medical School

"Stress management may reduce health problems linked to stress, which include cognitive problems and a higher risk for Alzheimer's disease and dementia[112]."

Managing stress might save your life and help you avoid dementia. A few recommendations:

- Meditation
- Exercise each day
- Eat a balanced wholefood diet
- Avoid people and activities that cause your stress

Take these and other natural steps to reduce your stress, improve your health, and increase your longevity.

Tobacco

Tobacco has killed more humans than all wars combined. For the killer weed, politicians and business people have always placed profit above public safety.

Using tobacco increases your risk of almost every disease on the planet, including Alzheimer's disease. Both smoking and secondhand smoke cause Alzheimer's[113].

Tobacco is a senseless habit that has killed more people than all wars combined.

"The chief preventable cause of death worldwide," says the World Alzheimer's Report[114].

> The annual global deaths due to tobacco are still expected to increase from the current six million, to eight million people by 2030. Cigarette smoking is causally related to a wide range of diseases 42 including many forms of cancer, cardiovascular disease and diabetes as well as increased risk of dyslipidaemia. The most prevalent dementia subtypes, vascular dementia (VaD) and Alzheimer's disease (AD), have been linked to underlying vascular mechanisms and neurovascular events.

Tobacco addiction makes a person crave and feel they cannot live without an immediate fix, but it destroys the body and mind.

Secondhand smoke also increases your risk for many diseases, so do not allow others to smoke in your presence, or in any establishment you live, work, or frequent.

How does Tobacco Increase Alzheimer's Risk?

Let's begin with a Columbia University study.

Columbia University Study Published in the US National Library of Medicine National Institutes of Health

A Columbia University study followed 1,138 dementia-free people in their seventies to determine if smoking tobacco elevates risks of Alzheimer's.

The researchers analyzed data from a northern Manhattan longitudinal study and found smoking and diabetes were the highest risk factors for Alzheimer's. They concluded: "Our results are consistent with the observation that smoking increases the risk of AD {Alzheimer's}[115]."

A University of San Francisco Review Published in the US National Library of Medicine National Institutes of Health

The University of San Francisco researchers reviewed several published studies on tobacco and nicotine. They compared smokers to nonsmokers[116].

The literature indicates that former/active smoking is related to a significantly increased risk for AD. Cigarette smoke/smoking is associated with AD neuropathology in preclinical models and humans. Smoking-related cerebral oxidative stress is a potential mechanism promoting AD pathophysiology and increased risk for AD.

The Observational University of California Study Published on Pub Med

A University of California observational studies found smokers carry a 79 percent greater risk of Alzheimer's than do nonsmokers[117].

World Health Organization

The World Health Organization claims smoking increases

one's chance of Alzheimer's by 45 percent[118].

Every credible organization I know lists tobacco as a risk for Alzheimer's and Posterior cortical atrophy. Nature and man have never built another killer like tobacco, as it kills millions each year, and leaves millions of others with one dementia, cancer, or some other devastating disease.

If you smoke, the best thing you can do for yourself and those around you is to quit. Among other health benefits, it will reduce your risk of Alzheimer's.

Prevention Measure 11

Do not smoke!

If you already smoke, quit! If you do not smoke, never start!

Do not use any tobacco products. No vaping. No cigarettes. No chewing tobacco. No snuff. No tobacco in any recreational form!

Type-2 Diabetes

According to the American Diabetes Association, 9.4 percent of Americans, over 30 million in total, have diabetes[119].

Let's review the global population.

The World Health Organization (WHO) reports that over 422 million people have Type-2 diabetes worldwide[120]. WHO lists Type-2 diabetes as the seventh leading cause of death worldwide, two behind Alzheimer's disease at number five[121].

Worldwide, a minimum of 371 million people has Type-2 diabetes.

Type-2 Diabetes is 100 percent Avoidable!

Type-2 diabetes is 100 percent avoidable, and fixable through diet, exercise, and weight management.

Before high blood sugar elevates enough to Type-2 Diabetes levels, there is a period called Hyperglycemia/high blood sugar/prediabetes.

Before we dive into Type-2 Diabetes, let's determine if prediabetes increases the risk of Alzheimer's.

High Blood Sugar/Hyperglycemia/Prediabetes

Hyperglycemia, meaning high blood sugar, but not high enough to rank as diabetes. For this discussion, we refer to it as prediabetes.

Several studies link high blood sugar levels and higher Alzheimer's risks, speeding and worsening the disease.

Let's begin with a German study that changed the way we view blood sugar and how the brain processes it.

Director of the drug discovery division at the German Center for Diabetes Research (DZD), Matthias Tschöp reported their findings[122]:

Our results showed for the first time that essential metabolic and behavioral processes are not regulated via neuronal cells alone and that other cell types in the brain, such as astrocytes, play a crucial role. This represents a paradigm shift and could help explain why it has been so difficult to find sufficiently efficient and save medicines for diabetes and obesity until now.

While other studies had discovered a link between high blood pressure and Alzheimer's, the German study might explain why. We now know much more is going on inside the brain than we thought when processing sugar.

Type-2 Diabetes

If prediabetes elevates the risks of Alzheimer's, Type-2 Diabetes is a bigger culprit. Type-2 diabetes, obesity, high blood pressure each to varying degrees the product of poor diets, and inadequate exercise.

An obese person has a higher risk of developing Type-2 diabetes and hypertension. The three diseases attack cells and damage the brain, heart, and blood flow.

Obesity, high blood pressure, and Type-2 diabetes is the perfect cocktail for strokes, heart disease, and the dementias, including Alzheimer's.

Studies confirming Type-2 Diabetes link to Alzheimer's

Scientists at the University of Cambridge teamed up with colleagues in Taiwan and Japan to follow 67,731 participants to study the connection. "Diabetes is associated with an increased risk of dementia[123]," reported Stephen Kritchevsky, Ph.D.

Early diagnosis and the correct medication can offset the risk. "The risk effect becomes weaker," said Kritchevsky said, "provided that participants take sulfonylureas or metformin rather than thiazolidinedione for a longer period."

Researchers in another longitudinal cohort study followed 824 older priests, brothers, and nuns in annual examinations over nine years. They concluded diabetes mellitus raised Alzheimer's risks and caused cognitive function decline in older persons[124]:

> *Diabetes mellitus was present in 127 (15.4%) of the participants. During a mean of 5.5 years of observation, 151 persons developed AD. In a proportional hazards model adjusted for age, sex, and educational level, those with diabetes mellitus had a 65% increase in the risk of developing AD compared with those without diabetes mellitus (hazard ratio, 1.65; 95% confidence interval, 1.10-2.47). In random effects models, diabetes mellitus was associated with lower levels of global cognition, episodic memory, semantic memory, working memory, and visuospatial ability at baseline. Diabetes mellitus was associated with a 44% greater rate of decline in perceptual speed (P = .02), but not in other cognitive systems.*

Most research confirms Type-2 diabetes increases risks to Alzheimer's by 50 to 65 percent.

How about when Diabetes Patients also experience Depression?

A University of Washington School of Medicine study focused on 19,239 diabetes patients to determine if diabetes and depression carried extra Alzheimer's risks. Wayne Katon, MD, Professor and Vice-Chair, Department of Psychiatry & Behavioral Sciences, reported their findings.

"Depression in patients with diabetes," said Katon, "with a substantively increased risk for development of dementia compared to those with diabetes alone[125]."

Depression compounds other diseases, including diabetes, hypertension, obesity, intensifying Alzheimer's risk factors.

134

Prevention Measure 12

Through bad habits, we cause most type-2 diabetes.

Our recommendations to avoid type-2 diabetes:

- A balanced wholefood diet
- Daily exercise
- Avoid sitting for longer than 25 minutes
- Do not drink alcohol

Once again, I reiterate researchers confirm the risk factors for typical Alzheimer's, but we need more research to confirm the same risk factors apply to posterior cortical atrophy. However, since posterior cortical atrophy develops AD, most or all should apply.

VI. BONUS SECTION

Whether diagnosed with dementia or preparing for a rainy day, there are basics everybody should consider.

This section focuses on steps dementia patients (all adults) should address, including forming a care team and understanding various therapy.

While written for dementia patients, I recommend every adult fulfill these tasks before you turn thirty. Waiting is our enemy for these two duties. Be prepared!

The section includes:

1. A starter to-do list for any adult diagnosed with a fatal disease such as dementia.
2. A care team plan.

Chapter 10: Starter To-do List for Somebody and Family once Diagnosed with Dementia.

Dementia patients, loved ones, and family must address several matters early in the disease, including care, financial decisions, living quarters, Living Will, and Power of Attorney.

While you have full or most of your cognitive skills, take care of the listed priorities before diagnosis or when diagnosed. Please do not consider the items covered in this section a complete care list, but a start you tailor to your needs.

Fail to cross these items off the list while you maintain your facilities causes much regret for patients and loved ones.

Your life is your ship, and for now, you remain the captain. Plan how your ship faces the coming storm and, when you can no longer captain the ship yourself, have it already determined who takes over the helm.

Now remains your last best chance to have a substantial say in your future.

Care

Family, loved ones, and dementia patients must make difficult decisions concerning if somebody can become the primary volunteer caregiver. While dementia patients do not require 24/7 care in the early stage, it becomes necessary in the middle to late stages.

Nobody can get through dementia without others providing years of caregiving. While rare dementias kill in months, most dementia patients live for 5-20 years, with dementia growing progressively worse.

Diagnosed with dementia or in perfect health, we all must ask ourselves who would take care of us if dementia or another devastating disorder struck, requiring long-term caregiving.

Most families cannot afford professional caregiving, and the government will not help until towards the end, so family and loved ones must.

In an ideal world, we ask ourselves these tough questions and have a plan in place should something happen. This benefits not only those diagnosed with dementia but also the heroic voluntary caregivers who will see them to the end.

Financial Decisions

There are significant financial decisions to make, and earlier, the better.

Find out how much your insurance covers and the amount you must pay. A kinder world would not burden dementia patients, nor their loved ones, with overwhelming medical care costs.

In the United States and most countries in the world, the majority of dementia costs fall on families.

How Much Does Dementia Cost the Average Family?

With no urine or blood test for most dementia types, neurologists must rely on imaging and other expensive tests, often not to diagnose dementia but to rule out other neurological disorders.

Under the best scenario, related tests, doctor visits saddle the average patient with tens of thousands of dollars in deductibles by the time the neurological team diagnoses them with dementia. For some, such as dementia with Lewy bodies, it might run much higher as it can take up to eighteen months or longer before doctors make a correct diagnosis.

Our health system tells the average person: "Sorry, you have dementia. Oh, by the way, there's the bill."

Doctors, medical professionals, hospitals, drug companies, and others involved in treating dementia must make a living. Even when we factor out overcharging and profiteering, treating dementia would remain expensive.

The average American family's health insurance has deteriorated for years, the premiums growing too high, the deductibles unaffordable, and too many not worth the paper its written, much less the monthly premiums.

Authorities estimate the average cost per dementia patient is $341,840, with families expected to cover 70 percent.

Such a disease becomes a hardship for not only the patient but also their family. The demands, financial and otherwise, on voluntary caregivers often is devastating. Make difficult financial decisions early.

Financial costs vary from one dementia to another and the treatment plan.

Living Quarters

While most dementia patients maintain independence in stage one, at some point, they require help with daily tasks. Will somebody move in with her or him? Does the patient move in with somebody else? Will it become necessary for him or her to move into an assisted living community in later stages? If so, what type?

The person diagnosed should gather loved ones and decide such matters in the beginning. Like somebody on a small island with a hurricane approaching, one must be diligent. While no man or woman can withstand such a storm, they still take precautions to protect themselves and their families.

In part because of financial considerations, most families care for the loved one in the home until symptoms grow critical. Whether a dementia patient ends up in a special needs living facility is not a matter of if, but at what point for those who have access.

No matter how much love, care, and attention a voluntary caregiver or loved ones provide a dementia patient, they are ill-equipped to provide for somebody in the disorder's final stretch.

Families without access do the best they can to provide comfort for the loved one but make no mistake, the patient and family benefit if a special needs facility takes over at some point.

Which type of facility depends on which dementia and symptoms. Some dementias cause more cognitive problems, while others greater affect motor skills, some visual, and a few dementias cause more language problems. In the end, many dementias are more alike than not, as the damage to the brain spreads to other areas. Still, depending on the symptoms, different care facilities might be better than others.

Ask your neurologist or local dementia organizations about local facilities trained for your particular type. Hopefully, you live at home and maintain a normal or semi-normal life for years, but have a facility selected when the end grows near.

Living Will

Not to be confused with a Last Will and Testament that distributes assets, a living will focus on medical decisions. NOLO defines a living will.

> *A living will – sometimes called a health care declaration -- is a document in which you describe the kind of health care you want to receive if you are incapacitated and cannot speak for yourself. It is often paired with a power of attorney for health care, in which you name an agent to make health care decisions on your behalf. Some states combine these two documents into one document called an 'advanced directive.'*

It is crucial to document the dementia patient's wishes while you maintain facilities to make such decisions.

Use the Living Will to direct physicians to follow your wishes on what care you receive now and in the future when you might not maintain your cognitive skills.

Specify end-of-life medical treatment.

NOLO recommends prioritizing life-prolonging medical care, food, and water if you become unconscious, and palliative care, which we soon address[126].

Distribute copies of your living will to loved ones, doctors, insurance providers, and all health care facilities.

Power of Attorney

The American Bar Association describes a power of attorney:

> *A power of attorney gives one or more persons the power to act on your behalf as your agent. The power may be limited to a particular activity, such as closing the sale of your home or be general in its application. The power may give temporary or permanent authority to act on your behalf. The power may take effect immediately, or only upon the occurrence of a future event, usually a determination that you are unable to act for yourself due to mental or physical disability. The latter is called a "springing" power of attorney. A power of attorney may be revoked, but most states require written notice of revocation to the person named to act for you[127].*

It is important to establish a medical power of attorney to empower a trusted loved one to make medical decisions when a patient becomes incapable. If you do not choose the right person, you can almost count on the wrong people making important decisions down the road.

If you're in early stages dementia and reading this, you likely can still think clearly, but this changes as the symptoms worsen. The only way to protect a dementia patient's wishes when they lose their cognitive decision-making is by naming a power of attorney in advance.

Once you name a power of attorney, cover some dos and don'ts. After all, you are trusting another person with your life. Like with your doctors, speak your mind while you can and let people know what you expect.

As NOLO pointed out, some states merge the living will and power of attorney into an advanced directive. Whether together or separate, I recommend all adults, and particularly those diagnosed with dementia draw up a medical living will and name a power of attorney.

The starter to-do list provides a starting point for dementia patients, families, and any adult.

Once diagnosed, both the person diagnosed and loved ones must unite and build your to-do list. Add whatever makes sense for you and your unique situation.

Let's next cover a few key members of a dementia care team.

Chapter 11: CARE TEAM

The National Institute on Aging recommends building a care team.

The team includes an art therapist, mental health counselor, occupational therapist, palliative care specialist, physical therapist, and a speech therapist[128].

Art therapist

The art therapist reduces stress by engaging the patient in music and other expressive arts.

Since dementia causes enormous anxiety and mood swings, art therapists use music and art to soothe patients and assist caregivers. Most everybody responds to music. Some pump our blood and makes us want to shake our bodies to the rhythm. Other music helps us focus and achieve maximum concentration.

Some music geared towards dementia patients relaxes and calms. Music is a godsend!

Art is not a task but a love affair. Some say within each of us is an artist starving to escape. Art therapists use music and art as a brilliant tool to treat dementia anxiety, attention decline, sleep problems, etc.

Mental health counselors

A neurological disorder, dementia attacks the brain and inhibits cognitive skills. Mental health counselors help patients and families plan for the future and cope with the shock, hurt, and pain resulting from the diagnosis.

Most individuals and families suffer chronic mental stress when doctors diagnose a member with dementia.

Find a mental health counselor trained in dementia.

Turn to their expertise and do not allow the neurological disorder to destroy the remaining quality of life for the patient, or respond as a family in a way where dementia destroys many lives by one sweeping event.

Occupational therapists

The occupational therapist helps patients bathe, dress, eat, and perform daily tasks.

We think of the routine daily tasks as second nature, and it is as long as the neurons, pathways, arteries, heart, and brain perform as normal. When suffering a stroke or neurological disorder like dementia, we quickly learn nothing is second nature anymore. Like a child, dementia patients often must relearn how to perform basic tasks.

Occupational therapists help patients remain independent and then semi-independent, as long as possible, extending the quality of life. An occupational therapist is instrumental in treating most dementias.

Palliative care specialist

The palliative care specialist minimizes symptoms from diagnosis to the end. You or a loved one need somebody who addresses symptoms as soon as they arise, so find a quality palliative care specialist.

They extend the quality of life and reduce suffering.

Physical therapists

Physical therapists help motors skills by leading patients through exercise.

Although dementia is known as a mental disorder, what affects the brain affects the body and vice versa. Find a physical therapist trained to work with your specific dementia.

If you've seen somebody suffering Parkinsonism or other neurological disorders affecting movement, you have an idea of the problems some dementias cause, even in the earliest stages.

A physical therapist helps maintain balance and strength, allowing a person to walk and move on their own. As dementia progresses, so does the physical therapist's importance.

Speech therapists

The speech therapist addresses speech and swallowing problems, issues present in early dementia symptoms for some types, and eventually becomes a problem for most dementias.

What is the value of verbalizing one's thoughts, understanding what a loved one says, and swallowing our food without choking or causing infection by sending it down the wrong pipe?

These are issues speech therapists excel. The ones I've observed are passionate about helping people retrain the mind to overcome aphasia and swallowing problems.

Find a speech (and other types of) therapist trained in treating your specific type of dementia. These different listed therapists can minimize the long nightmare following a dementia diagnosis.

Chapter 12: LETTER TO CONGRESS

DEAR U.S. CONGRESS, NATIONS OF THE WORLD, & WEALTHY HUMANS

We call on the United States and the governments of the world to spend less on war and walls and more on Alzheimer's and dementia research.

If aliens were attacking us from another planet, I presume the nations of the world would unite against a common enemy. That is what I propose now.

The enemy I refer to does not come from another planet but threatens humans no less. Alzheimer's and dementia strike an American every 68 seconds and somebody worldwide every 30 seconds.

The nations of the world can save millions of lives and billions of dollars.

We need necessary funding to:

1. Discover the exact cause (s) of Alzheimer's and other dementias.
2. Develop accurate testing for Alzheimer's and other dementias.
3. Develop a vaccine to wipe out Alzheimer's and other dementias like we did polio.

Alzheimer's and dementia grow at a rate that will destroy the economies of most countries if we do not become more proactive.

We can save trillions of dollars for future generations if we invest now in discovering the exact cause (s), a vaccine to prevent it from happening, and other steps to defeat this horrifying disease.

Alzheimer's and other dementias threaten every family in all nations.

We can do little for those with late-stage dementia, but the proposed steps might save millions of lives and trillions of dollars by diagnosing the different dementias early and treating them before they do significant damage.

Beller Health calls on politicians, corporations, and wealthy individuals to step forward to help win the war against dementia.

●

CONCLUSION

Thank you for reading this book. We covered a good amount of material.

Dementia is a cruel neurological disorder that robs people of their personalities, executive skills, memories, talents, language, voice, motor capabilities, and all that makes us individual humans.

Alzheimer's and Dementia

Although Alzheimer's disease (AD) is the most prevalent, we learned AD is to dementia what China is to Asia. Alzheimer's represents 60-80% of dementia, but 19 dementia types account for 99 percent.

Dementia Spares No Demographic

Dementia's reputation is known as an old folk's disease but strikes people all ages. Most dementia is not genetic, although certain types such as Huntington's disease are 100% familial.

Most Dementia is Incurable

Most dementia is incurable, but—if caught early enough—neurosurgeons can treat and sometimes reverse normal pressure hydrocephalus.

Dementia Prevalence

The first section focused on dementia as a general category. We learned 850,000 people in the UK have dementia, compared to 5.8 Americans and 50 million people worldwide.

Dementia Categories

We divided the 19 dementias into six categories:

- Lewy Body/Parkinsonism related dementias
- Alzheimer's related dementias
- Frontotemporal lobar degeneration related dementias
- Primary progressive aphasia related dementias
- Vascular dementias
- Other dementias

19 Dementia Types

Lewy Body/Parkinsonism Related Dementias

1. *Dementia with Lewy Bodies*
2. *Parkinson's Disease Dementia*
3. Corticobasal Syndrome

Alzheimer's Related Dementias

4. Typical Alzheimer's Disease
5. *Posterior Cortical Atrophy*
6. *Down Syndrome with Alzheimer's*
7. *Limbic-predominant Age-related TDP-43 Encephalopathy (LATE)*
8. Early-onset Alzheimer's

Frontotemporal Lobar Degeneration Related Dementias

9. *Behavioral Variant Frontotemporal Dementia*
10. Progressive Supranuclear Palsy

Primary Progressive Aphasia Related Dementias

11. *Nonfluent Primary Progressive Aphasia (nfvPPA)*

12. Logopenic Progressive Aphasia (LPA)

Vascular Dementia

13. *Cortical Vascular Dementia*
14. *Binswanger Disease*

Other Dementias

15. *Normal Pressure Hydrocephalus*
16. *Huntington's Disease*
17. *Korsakoff Syndrome*
18. *Creutzfeldt-Jakob Disease*
19. Amyotrophic Lateral Sclerosis

We examined the prevalence, costs, subtypes, symptoms, stages, and risk factors for Posterior Cortical Atrophy.

THE END

Of

POSTERIOR CORTICAL ATROPHY

THANK YOU FOR READING

Thank you for reading the entire book. While this is not a literary work to enjoy, I hope you gained useful knowledge of posterior cortical atrophy.

If you benefitted from this book, please take a moment to share your thoughts in a review. Reader reviews help other readers make educated decisions about this book before purchasing.

Book Review link for Posterior Cortical Atrophy

or

https://www.amazon.com/dp/product/B07YZMQJ1X

Look for annual updates to my health books, as I follow new studies and add any helpful information I find. Health and fitness are top priorities, and the heart and brain are my specialties.

I hope you develop the habits suggested in this book. Good luck on your health journey. Live long and prosper, my friend.

All the best,

Jerry Beller & Beller Health

BELLER HEALTH BOOKS

Beller Health Research Institute specializes in the heart and brain, and published the following Jerry Beller book series:

- Arrhythmia Series
- Vascular Disease Series
- 2020 Dementia Overview Series
- 19 Dementia Types Series

Please continue to view the books in each series.

Dementia Types, Symptoms, Stages, & Risk Factors Series

This book series is the first to cover each of the 19 primary dementia types.

2020 Dementia Overview Series

Whereas in the *Dementia Types, Symptoms, Stages, and Risk Factors* series, each book covers a different dementia type, this series focuses on groups of dementias.

1. Dementia Types, Symptoms, & Stages
2. *Lewy Body/Parkinsonism Dementias*
3. *Vascular Dementia*
4. *Frontotemporal Dementia (FTD)*
5. Alzheimer's Related Dementias
6. *Prevent or Slow Dementia*

Other Beller Health Books

You can view or purchase all Beller Health Books on Amazon at the following web address:

https://amzn.to/2TpDr8e

ABOUT THE AUTHOR

Jerry Beller is the lead author and researcher at Beller Medical Research Institute. Beller distinguished himself three times in the medical world by being the first to write and publish books on particular dementia fields.

He wrote the first book covering all 15 primary dementia types, which he since expanded to cover nineteen. Beller followed this accomplishment by writing a book on each dementia type. He broke medical ground a third time when he published the first book on the new dementia category LATE.

When the world struggled to grasp the difference between Alzheimer's disease and China, Beller explained:

Alzheimer's is only one dementia, much like China is only one country in Asia. Just as we do not want to ignore the other countries in Asia because China is the largest, nor do we want to ignore the less prevalent dementia types.

Despite his accomplishments, he remains humble. "Until we win the dementia war, I've no reason to celebrate," Beller said. "If we win the war during my lifetime, I will celebrate with a few hundred brothers and sisters around the world who share my passion. Until then, we have too much work left to worry about accolades and legacies."

When not researching dementia, Jerry enjoys life with his wife of thirty-plus years, Nicola, and their two children.

Visit Jerry Beller:

https://bellerhealth.com

*1 'What Is Dementia?', Alzheimer's Disease and Dementia
<https://alz.org/alzheimers-dementia/what-is-dementia> [accessed 18
September 2019].*

*2 'What Is Dementia? Symptoms, Types, and Diagnosis', National
Institute on Aging <https://www.nia.nih.gov/health/what-dementia-
symptoms-types-and-diagnosis> [accessed 18 September 2019].*

3 'What Is Dementia?', *Alzheimer's Society*
<https://www.alzheimers.org.uk/about-dementia/types-dementia/what-
dementia> [accessed 18 September 2019].

4 'Dementia' <https://www.who.int/news-room/fact-
sheets/detail/dementia> [accessed 18 September 2019].

5 'Risk Factors' <https://stanfordhealthcare.org/medical-
conditions/brain-and-nerves/dementia/risk-factors.html> [accessed 20
September 2019].

6 W. M. van der Flier and P. Scheltens, 'Epidemiology and Risk
Factors of Dementia', *Journal of Neurology, Neurosurgery & Psychiatry*,
76.suppl 5 (2005), v2–7 <https://doi.org/10.1136/jnnp.2005.082867>.

7 Kent Allen, 'Dementia Rates to Grow for African Americans,
Hispanics', *AARP* <http://www.aarp.org/health/dementia/info-
2018/dementia-alzheimer-cases-grow-nonwhites.html> [accessed 20
September 2019].

8 Elizabeth Rose Mayeda and others, 'Inequalities in Dementia
Incidence between Six Racial and Ethnic Groups over 14 Years', *Alzheimer's
& Dementia: The Journal of the Alzheimer's Association*, 12.3 (2016), 216–
24 <https://doi.org/10.1016/j.jalz.2015.12.007>.

9 'African Americans at Higher Dementia Risk than Other Racial
Groups', *Reuters*, 10 March 2016 <https://www.reuters.com/article/us-
health-dementia-race-u-s-idUSKCN0WC2X5> [accessed 20 September
2019].

10 Steve Ford, 'Likelihood of Dementia "Higher among Black Ethnic
Groups"', *Nursing Times*, 2018
<https://www.nursingtimes.net/news/research-and-innovation/likelihood-
of-dementia-higher-among-black-ethnic-groups-08-08-2018/> [accessed
21 September 2019].

11 'Dementia' <https://www.who.int/news-room/fact-
sheets/detail/dementia> [accessed 21 September 2019].

12 'Women and Alzheimer's', *Alzheimer's Disease and Dementia* <https://alz.org/alzheimers-dementia/what-is-alzheimers/women-and-alzheimer-s> [accessed 21 September 2019].

13 'Dementia Facts', *Dementia Consortium* <https://www.dementiaconsortium.org/dementia-facts/> [accessed 21 September 2019].

14 'Dementia' <https://www.who.int/news-room/fact-sheets/detail/dementia> [accessed 21 September 2019].

15 'Why Is Dementia Different for Women?', *Alzheimer's Society* <https://www.alzheimers.org.uk/blog/why-dementia-different-women> [accessed 21 September 2019].

16 Jessica L. Podcasy and C. Neill Epperson, 'Considering Sex and Gender in Alzheimer Disease and Other Dementias', *Dialogues in Clinical Neuroscience*, 18.4 (2016), 437–46 <https://www.ncbi.nlm.nih.gov/pmc/articles/PMC5286729/> [accessed 21 September 2019].

17 'WHO | Life Expectancy', *WHO* <http://www.who.int/gho/mortality_burden_disease/life_tables/situation_trends_text/en/> [accessed 21 September 2019].

18 'Products - Data Briefs - Number 328 - November 2018', 2019 <https://www.cdc.gov/nchs/products/databriefs/db328.htm> [accessed 21 September 2019].

19 Jacqui Thornton, 'WHO Report Shows That Women Outlive Men Worldwide', *BMJ*, 365 (2019), l1631 <https://doi.org/10.1136/bmj.l1631>.

20 'Why Do Women Live Longer Than Men?', *Time* <https://time.com/5538099/why-do-women-live-longer-than-men/> [accessed 21 September 2019].

21 'Dementia' <https://www.who.int/news-room/fact-sheets/detail/dementia> [accessed 20 September 2019].

22 'Alzheimer's Disease: Facts & Figures', *BrightFocus Foundation*, 2015 <https://www.brightfocus.org/alzheimers/article/alzheimers-disease-facts-figures> [accessed 4 September 2019].

23 'Facts for the Media', *Alzheimer's Society* <https://www.alzheimers.org.uk/about-us/news-and-media/facts-media> [accessed 20 September 2019].

24 'Countries With The Highest Rates Of Deaths From Dementia',

WorldAtlas <https://www.worldatlas.com/articles/countries-with-the-highest-rates-of-deaths-from-dementia.html> [accessed 20 September 2019].

[25] 'World Alzheimer Report 2018 - The State of the Art of Dementia Research: New Frontiers', *NEW FRONTIERS*, 48.

[26] 'ALZHEIMERS/DEMENTIA DEATH RATE BY COUNTRY', *World Life Expectancy* <https://www.worldlifeexpectancy.com/cause-of-death/alzheimers-dementia/by-country/> [accessed 24 September 2019].

[27] 'Alzheimer Europe - Research - European Collaboration on Dementia - Cost of Dementia - Regional/National Cost of Illness Estimates' <https://www.alzheimer-europe.org/Research/European-Collaboration-on-Dementia/Cost-of-dementia/Regional-National-cost-of-illness-estimates> [accessed 26 September 2019].

[28] 'Publications | NATSEM' <https://www.natsem.canberra.edu.au/publications/?publication=economic-cost-of-dementia-in-australia-2016-2056> [accessed 22 September 2019].

[29] 'Dementia UK Report', *Alzheimer's Society* <https://www.alzheimers.org.uk/about-us/policy-and-influencing/dementia-uk-report> [accessed 22 September 2019].

[30] 'Dementia Statistics – U.S. & Worldwide Stats', *BrainTest*, 2015 <https://braintest.com/dementia-stats-u-s-worldwide/> [accessed 23 September 2019].

[31] 'Newsroom | Northwestern Mutual - 2018 C.A.R.E. Study', *Newsroom | Northwestern Mutual* <https://news.northwesternmutual.com/2018-care-study> [accessed 22 September 2019].

[32] 'ALZHEIMERS/DEMENTIA DEATH RATE BY COUNTRY'.

[33] 'Alzheimer Europe - Research - European Collaboration on Dementia - Cost of Dementia - Regional/National Cost of Illness Estimates'.

[34] 'Publications | NATSEM'.

[35] 'Dementia UK Report'.

[36] 'Dementia Statistics – U.S. & Worldwide Stats'.

[37] 'Posterior Cortical Atrophy', *Memory and Aging Center* <https://memory.ucsf.edu/dementia/posterior-cortical-atrophy> [accessed 13 November 2019].

[38] 'Posterior Cortical Atrophy', *Memory and Aging Center*

<https://memory.ucsf.edu/dementia/posterior-cortical-atrophy> [accessed 13 November 2019].

39 'Posterior Cortical Atrophy', *Memory and Aging Center* <https://memory.ucsf.edu/dementia/posterior-cortical-atrophy> [accessed 26 July 2019].

40 INSERM US14-- ALL RIGHTS RESERVED, 'Orphanet: Posterior Cortical Atrophy' <https://www.orpha.net/consor/cgi-bin/OC_Exp.php?Lng=GB&Expert=54247> [accessed 28 July 2019].

41 'Posterior Cortical Atrophy', *Alzheimer's Society* <https://www.alzheimers.org.uk/about-dementia/types-dementia/Posterior-cortical-atrophy> [accessed 26 July 2019].

42 'Posterior Cortical Atrophy'.

43 Sebastian J. Crutch and others, 'Consensus Classification of Posterior Cortical Atrophy', *Alzheimer's & Dementia*, 13.8 (2017), 870–84 <https://doi.org/10.1016/j.jalz.2017.01.014>.

44 'Global.Pdf' <https://www.fhca.org/members/qi/clinadmin/global.pdf> [accessed 28 July 2019].

45 'Stages of Alzheimer's', *Alzheimer's Disease and Dementia* <https://alz.org/alzheimers-dementia/stages> [accessed 28 July 2019].

46 'Alzheimer's Disease Center', *NYU Langone Health* <https://med.nyu.edu/departments-institutes/neurology/divisions-centers/center-cognitive-neurology/alzheimers-disease-center> [accessed 28 July 2019].

47 Crutch and others.

48 '2016-Facts-and-Figures.Pdf' <https://www.alz.org/documents_custom/2016-facts-and-figures.pdf> [accessed 18 February 2018].

49 Rita Guerreiro and Jose Bras, 'The Age Factor in Alzheimer's Disease', *Genome Medicine*, 7 (2015) <https://doi.org/10.1186/s13073-015-0232-5>.

50 'Alcohol and Tobacco - Alcohol Alert No. 39-1998' <https://pubs.niaaa.nih.gov/publications/aa39.htm> [accessed 7 December 2018].

51 Christi A. Patten, John E. Martin, and Neville Owen,

'Can Psychiatric and Chemical Dependency Treatment Units Be Smoke Free?', *Journal of Substance Abuse Treatment*, 13.2 (1996), 107–18 <https://doi.org/10.1016/0740-5472(96)00040-2>.

[52] 'CDC - Fact Sheets-Alcohol Use And Health - Alcohol', 2018 <https://www.cdc.gov/alcohol/fact-sheets/alcohol-use.htm> [accessed 7 December 2018].

[53] 'WHO | Alcohol', *WHO* <https://www.who.int/substance_abuse/facts/alcohol/en/> [accessed 7 December 2018].

[54] 'CDC - Frequently Asked Questions - Alcohol', 2017 <https://www.cdc.gov/alcohol/faqs.htm> [accessed 19 February 2018].

[55] 'Alcohol-Related Brain Damage', *Alzheimer's Society* <https://www.alzheimers.org.uk/about-dementia/types-dementia/alcohol-related-brain-damage> [accessed 7 December 2018].

[56] Paul R. Albert, 'Why Is Depression More Prevalent in Women?', *Journal of Psychiatry & Neuroscience□ : JPN*, 40.4 (2015), 219–21 <https://doi.org/10.1503/jpn.150205>.

[57] 'Depression in Women: Understanding the Gender Gap', *Mayo Clinic* <https://www.mayoclinic.org/diseases-conditions/depression/in-depth/depression/art-20047725> [accessed 8 December 2018].

[58] Archana Singh-Manoux and others, 'Trajectories of Depressive Symptoms Before Diagnosis of Dementia: A 28-Year Follow-up Study', *JAMA Psychiatry*, 74.7 (2017), 712–18 <https://doi.org/10.1001/jamapsychiatry.2017.0660>.

[59] Breno S. Diniz and others, 'Late-Life Depression and Risk of Vascular Dementia and Alzheimer's Disease: Systematic Review and Meta-Analysis of Community-Based Cohort Studies', *The British Journal of Psychiatry*, 202.5 (2013), 329–35

<https://doi.org/10.1192/bjp.bp.112.118307>.

60 'Alzheimer's or Depression: Could It Be Both?', *Mayo Clinic* <https://www.mayoclinic.org/diseases-conditions/alzheimers-disease/in-depth/alzheimers/art-20048362> [accessed 7 December 2018].

61 Amy L. Byers and Kristine Yaffe, 'Depression and Risk of Developing Dementia', *Nature Reviews. Neurology*, 7.6 (2011), 323–31 <https://doi.org/10.1038/nrneurol.2011.60>.

62 Raymond L. Ownby and others, 'Depression and Risk for Alzheimer Disease', *Archives of General Psychiatry*, 63.5 (2006), 530–38 <https://doi.org/10.1001/archpsyc.63.5.530>.

63 'Alzheimer's Disease - Symptoms and Causes', *Mayo Clinic* <http://www.mayoclinic.org/diseases-conditions/alzheimers-disease/symptoms-causes/syc-20350447> [accessed 19 February 2018].

64 'Alzheimer's Disease & Down Syndrome', *NDSS* <https://www.ndss.org/resources/alzheimers/> [accessed 4 December 2018].

65 'Aging-and-Down-Syndrome.Pdf' <http://www.ndss.org/wp-content/uploads/2017/11/Aging-and-Down-Syndrome.pdf> [accessed 4 December 2018].

66 'NDSS_Guidebook_FINAL.Pdf' <http://www.ndss.org/wp-content/uploads/2017/11/NDSS_Guidebook_FINAL.pdf> [accessed 9 December 2018].

67 'Alzheimer's Disease & Down Syndrome', *NDSS* <https://www.ndss.org/resources/alzheimers/> [accessed 9 December 2018].

68 'How Does Alzheimer's Affect Women and Men Differently? | Cognitive Vitality | Alzheimer's Drug Discovery

Foundation' <https://www.alzdiscovery.org/cognitive-vitality/blog/how-does-alzheimers-affect-women-and-men-differently> [accessed 7 December 2018].

⁶⁹ Martin Prince and others, 'Recent Global Trends in the Prevalence and Incidence of Dementia, and Survival with Dementia', *Alzheimer's Research & Therapy*, 8.1 (2016), 23 <https://doi.org/10.1186/s13195-016-0188-8>.

⁷⁰ Jessica L. Podcasy and C. Neill Epperson, 'Considering Sex and Gender in Alzheimer Disease and Other Dementias', *Dialogues in Clinical Neuroscience*, 18.4 (2016), 437–46 <https://www.ncbi.nlm.nih.gov/pmc/articles/PMC5286729/> [accessed 9 December 2018].

⁷¹ 'Scientists Shed New Light on Gender Differences in Alzheimer's', *BrightFocus Foundation*, 2017 <https://www.brightfocus.org/alzheimers/news/scientists-shed-new-light-gender-differences-alzheimers> [accessed 9 December 2018].

⁷² 'Assessing Risk for Alzheimer's Disease', *National Institute on Aging* <http://www.nia.nih.gov/health/assessing-risk-alzheimers-disease> [accessed 19 February 2018].

⁷³ Lars Bertram and Rudolph E. Tanzi, 'Thirty Years of Alzheimer's Disease Genetics: The Implications of Systematic Meta-Analyses', *Nature Reviews Neuroscience*, 9.10 (2008), 768–78 <https://doi.org/10.1038/nrn2494>.

⁷⁴ 'Early-Onset Alzheimer's: Symptoms, Diagnosis, and Treatment', *Medical News Today* <https://www.medicalnewstoday.com/articles/315247.php> [accessed 9 December 2018].

⁷⁵ 'Alzheimer's Disease Genetics Fact Sheet', *National Institute on Aging* <https://www.nia.nih.gov/health/alzheimers-disease-

genetics-fact-sheet> [accessed 9 December 2018].

76 'Scientists Fix Genetic Risk Factor for Alzheimer's Disease in Human Brain Cells: New Insights into How a Gene Causes Damage Could Impact Future Drug Development', *ScienceDaily* <https://www.sciencedaily.com/releases/2018/04/1804091 12559.htm> [accessed 9 December 2018].

77 Kenny Walter, 'Scientists Identify Genetic Risk Factor for Alzheimer's', *Research & Development*, 2018 <https://www.rdmag.com/article/2018/04/scientists-identify-genetic-risk-factor-alzheimers> [accessed 10 December 2018].

78 Chengzhong Wang and others, 'Gain of Toxic Apolipoprotein E4 Effects in Human IPSC-Derived Neurons Is Ameliorated by a Small-Molecule Structure Corrector', *Nature Medicine*, 24.5 (2018), 647 <https://doi.org/10.1038/s41591-018-0004-z>.

79 Emer R. McGrath and others, 'Blood Pressure from Mid- to Late Life and Risk of Incident Dementia', *Neurology*, 89.24 (2017), 2447–54 <https://doi.org/10.1212/WNL.0000000000004741>.

80 'AAN' <https://www.aan.com/PressRoom/Home/PressRelease/16 60> [accessed 10 December 2018].

81 'Hypertension Highlights 2017', 22.

82 'More than 100 Million Americans Have High Blood Pressure, AHA Says', *Www.Heart.Org* <https://www.heart.org/en/news/2018/05/01/more-than-100-million-americans-have-high-blood-pressure-aha-says> [accessed 10 December 2018].

83 'WHO | Raised Blood Pressure', *WHO* <https://www.who.int/gho/ncd/risk_factors/blood_pressur e_prevalence_text/en/> [accessed 10 December 2018].

[84] 'Risk Factors | Alzheimer Society of Canada' <http://alzheimer.ca/en/Home/About-dementia/Alzheimer-s-disease/Risk-factors> [accessed 19 February 2018].

[85] 'Frequent Brain Stimulation In Old Age Reduces Risk Of Alzheimer's Disease', *ScienceDaily* <https://www.sciencedaily.com/releases/2007/06/0706271 61810.htm> [accessed 10 December 2018].

[86] Robert S. Wilson and others, 'Participation in Cognitively Stimulating Activities and Risk of Incident Alzheimer Disease', *JAMA*, 287.6 (2002), 742–48 <https://doi.org/10.1001/jama.287.6.742>.

[87] Panagiota Mistridis and others, 'Use It or Lose It! Cognitive Activity as a Protec-Tive Factor for Cognitive Decline Associated with Alzheimer's Disease', *Swiss Medical Weekly*, 147.0910 (2017) <https://doi.org/10.4414/smw.2017.14407>.

[88] '151-11-1064.Pdf' <https://watermark.silverchair.com/151-11-1064.pdf?token=

AQECAHi208BE49Ooan9kkhW_Ercy7Dm
3ZL_9Cf3qfKAc485ysgAAAlQwggJQBgkqhkiG9w0BBwaggg
JBMIICPQIBADCCAjYGCSqGSIb3DQEHATAeBglghkgBZQ
MEAS4wEQQMDIjEhY8xDH0-DMCPAgEQgIICB3lWtR5-
EpPRdmA3Ebh8sg0QeEDNQs8nFCJodObkuPlXhq6eQVjEs
E37NB6p4IndTkk_XqqVhAy2zDayOp5eMQZF6yAwZyDlVP
VszX4tIQPi5_ooPFbW6ODRDoBAdvzPFfuUJzv0aUv9prwm
h_ovV4p-
1cpp1MGn6smPZSXkq1CkZL9E3Luk4rhQ_tkMjSH4e9yMiP
9d2EenyAHW8_Wk4LraH_NXpgP6usnc9cBRAmBQziNcok
wnOOyNGpSBCVpVPD7oqJZBqdNBS5xdyRhBt30_2T7Prf5
cC9UkAZaGXfLvFkzJSz5X4tSFzY3TScQZBScgQTf97PrJ8Zo
MmedCMVofjGmXkAmyvD2nlwlUptOKkEyiOS9LSMPAqcv
RNb-EwHJ9ZTczj6l2deeuQetp2721IqB-
93FzhE5ZXRhHx9OPQwnpzeyfTuxK3U19-

957bYxZjJTYHiURrk3d4XLr4HB0BptwTN0qKpYquitYouA LtAprPH9oeIo_v5OyY2Gd39ZG1BbxkY-fy_SQw_y2Fod7CypRFZdBWQdAmnwP-xBPGOuqtM3R2V2vDj6UmU44-9-T8Aqh6Ovd5_OfVqOlVrgkGIZQfahgGHAfCWQQNrf9N8Y1 gUQNB02EZNmYrAjTkRv75ThvMsyk2KwPcPhU_7CRvZkE uissHgBs_3A_vuVYevnkRAX29Q> [accessed 10 December 2018].

⁸⁹ 'Low Education Level Linked To Alzheimer's, Study Shows', *ScienceDaily* <https://www.sciencedaily.com/releases/2007/10/071001172855.htm> [accessed 10 December 2018].

⁹⁰ Rachel A Whitmer and others, 'Obesity in Middle Age and Future Risk of Dementia: A 27 Year Longitudinal Population Based Study', *BMJ□: British Medical Journal*, 330.7504 (2005), 1360 <https://doi.org/10.1136/bmj.38446.466238.E0>.

⁹¹ Louis A. Profenno, Anton P. Porsteinsson, and Stephen V. Faraone, 'Meta-Analysis of Alzheimer's Disease Risk with Obesity, Diabetes, and Related Disorders', *Biological Psychiatry*, 67.6 (2010), 505–12 <https://doi.org/10.1016/j.biopsych.2009.02.013>.

⁹² Rachel A Whitmer and others, 'Obesity in Middle Age and Future Risk of Dementia: A 27 Year Longitudinal Population Based Study', *BMJ□: British Medical Journal*, 330.7504 (2005), 1360 <https://doi.org/10.1136/bmj.38446.466238.E0>.

⁹³ Miia Kivipelto and others, 'Obesity and Vascular Risk Factors at Midlife and the Risk of Dementia and Alzheimer Disease', *Archives of Neurology*, 62.10 (2005), 1556–60 <https://doi.org/10.1001/archneur.62.10.1556>.

⁹⁴ Nikolaos Scarmeas and others, 'Physical Activity, Diet, and Risk of Alzheimer Disease', *JAMA*, 302.6 (2009),

627–37 <https://doi.org/10.1001/jama.2009.1144>.

[95] Yves Rolland, Gabor Abellan van Kan, and Bruno Vellas, 'Physical Activity and Alzheimer's Disease: From Prevention to Therapeutic Perspectives', *Journal of the American Medical Directors Association*, 9.6 (2008), 390–405 <https://doi.org/10.1016/j.jamda.2008.02.007>.

[96] WEI-WEI CHEN, XIA ZHANG, and WEN-JUAN HUANG, 'Role of Physical Exercise in Alzheimer's Disease', *Biomedical Reports*, 4.4 (2016), 403–7 <https://doi.org/10.3892/br.2016.607>.

[97] Virva Hyttinen and others, 'Risk Factors for Initiation of Potentially Inappropriate Medications in Community-Dwelling Older Adults with and without Alzheimer's Disease', *Drugs & Aging*, 34.1 (2017), 67–77 <https://doi.org/10.1007/s40266-016-0415-9>.

[98] Beverly Merz, 'Benzodiazepine Use May Raise Risk of Alzheimer's Disease', *Harvard Health Blog*, 2014 <https://www.health.harvard.edu/blog/benzodiazepine-use-may-raise-risk-alzheimers-disease-201409107397> [accessed 19 February 2018].

[99] Harvard Health Publishing, 'Two Types of Drugs You May Want to Avoid for the Sake of Your Brain', *Harvard Health* <https://www.health.harvard.edu/mind-and-mood/two-types-of-drugs-you-may-want-to-avoid-for-the-sake-of-your-brain> [accessed 11 December 2018].

[100] Kathryn Richardson and others, 'Anticholinergic Drugs and Risk of Dementia: Case-Control Study', *BMJ*, 361 (2018), k1315 <https://doi.org/10.1136/bmj.k1315>.

[101] 'Worst Pills' <https://www.worstpills.org/includes/page.cfm?op_id=459> [accessed 11 December 2018].

[102] 'Mayo Clinic Q and A: Impaired Sleep and Risk of Dementia', *Https://Newsnetwork.Mayoclinic.Org*

<https://newsnetwork.mayoclinic.org/discussion/mayo-clinic-q-and-a-impaired-sleep-and-risk-of-dementia/> [accessed 11 December 2018].

[103] Ram A. Sharma and others, 'Obstructive Sleep Apnea Severity Affects Amyloid Burden in Cognitively Normal Elderly. A Longitudinal Study', *American Journal of Respiratory and Critical Care Medicine*, 197.7 (2017), 933–43 <https://doi.org/10.1164/rccm.201704-0704OC>.

[104] Weihong Pan and Abba J. Kastin, 'Can Sleep Apnea Cause Alzheimer's Disease?', *Neuroscience & Biobehavioral Reviews*, 47 (2014), 656–69 <https://doi.org/10.1016/j.neubiorev.2014.10.019>.

[105] Kristine Yaffe and others, 'Sleep-Disordered Breathing, Hypoxia, and Risk of Mild Cognitive Impairment and Dementia in Older Women', *JAMA*, 306.6 (2011), 613–19 <https://doi.org/10.1001/jama.2011.1115>.

[106] BarneysMusicIsGood, *Bobby McFerrin - Don't Worry Be Happy* <https://www.youtube.com/watch?v=yv-Fk1PwVeU> [accessed 22 February 2018].

[107] Sami Piirainen and others, 'Psychosocial Stress on Neuroinflammation and Cognitive Dysfunctions in Alzheimer's Disease: The Emerging Role for Microglia?', *Neuroscience & Biobehavioral Reviews*, 77 (2017), 148–64 <https://doi.org/10.1016/j.neubiorev.2017.01.046>.

[108] 'Do Beta-Amyloids Cause Alzheimers? | Science 2.0', 2014 <https://www.science20.com/news/do_beta_amyloids_cause_alzheimers> [accessed 11 December 2018].

[109] Matthew A. Stults-Kolehmainen and Rajita Sinha, 'The Effects of Stress on Physical Activity and Exercise', *Sports Medicine (Auckland, N.Z.)*, 44.1 (2014), 81–121 <https://doi.org/10.1007/s40279-013-0090-5>.

[110] Linda Mah, Claudia Szabuniewicz, and Alexandra J.

Fiocco, 'Can Anxiety Damage the Brain?', *Current Opinion in Psychiatry*, 29.1 (2016), 56–63 <https://doi.org/10.1097/YCO.0000000000000223>.

[111] 'AAN'.

[112] Harvard Health Publishing, 'Protect Your Brain from Stress', *Harvard Health* <https://www.health.harvard.edu/mind-and-mood/protect-your-brain-from-stress> [accessed 11 December 2018].

[113] Erin K. Saito and others, 'Smoking History and Alzheimer's Disease Risk in a Community-Based Clinic Population', *Journal of Education and Health Promotion*, 6 (2017) <https://doi.org/10.4103/jehp.jehp_45_15>.

[114] 'WorldAlzheimerReport2014.Pdf' <https://www.alz.co.uk/research/WorldAlzheimerReport2014.pdf> [accessed 7 December 2018].

[115] Jose Luchsinger and others, 'Aggregation of Vascular Risk Factors and Risk of Incident Alzheimer's Disease', *Neurology*, 65.4 (2005), 545–51 <https://doi.org/10.1212/01.wnl.0000172914.08967.dc>.

[116] Timothy C. Durazzo, Niklas Mattsson, and Michael W. Weiner, 'Smoking and Increased Alzheimer's Disease Risk: A Review of Potential Mechanisms', *Alzheimer's & Dementia□: The Journal of the Alzheimer's Association*, 10.3 0 (2014), S122–45 <https://doi.org/10.1016/j.jalz.2014.04.009>.

[117] Deborah E. Barnes and Kristine Yaffe, 'The Projected Effect of Risk Factor Reduction on Alzheimer's Disease Prevalence', *The Lancet. Neurology*, 10.9 (2011), 819–28 <https://doi.org/10.1016/S1474-4422(11)70072-2>.

[118] 'WHO_NMH_PND_CIC_TKS_14.1_eng.Pdf' <http://apps.who.int/iris/bitstream/handle/10665/128041/WHO_NMH_PND_CIC_TKS_14.1_eng.pdf?sequence=1> [accessed 11 December 2018].

[119] American Diabetes Association 2451 Crystal Drive, Suite 900 Arlington, and Va 22202 1-800-Diabetes, 'Statistics About Diabetes', *American Diabetes Association* <http://www.diabetes.org/diabetes-basics/statistics/> [accessed 8 December 2018].

[120] 'Diabetes' <https://www.who.int/news-room/fact-sheets/detail/diabetes> [accessed 8 December 2018].

[121] 'The Top 10 Causes of Death' <https://www.who.int/news-room/fact-sheets/detail/the-top-10-causes-of-death> [accessed 8 December 2018].

[122] 'Schalter Für Zuckertransport Ins Gehirn Entdeckt' <https://www.tum.de/en/about-tum/news/press-releases/detail/article/33322/> [accessed 6 December 2018].

[123] Chin Cheng and others, 'Type 2 Diabetes and Antidiabetic Medications in Relation to Dementia Diagnosis', *The Journals of Gerontology: Series A*, 69.10 (2014), 1299–1305 <https://doi.org/10.1093/gerona/glu073>.

[124] Zoe Arvanitakis and others, 'Diabetes Mellitus and Risk of Alzheimer Disease and Decline in Cognitive Function', *Archives of Neurology*, 61.5 (2004), 661–66 <https://doi.org/10.1001/archneur.61.5.661>.

[125] Wayne Katon and others, 'Depression Increases Risk of Dementia in Patients with Type 2 Diabetes: The Diabetes & Aging Study', *Archives of General Psychiatry*, 69.4 (2012), 410–17 <https://doi.org/10.1001/archgenpsychiatry.2011.154>.

[126] Betsy Simmons Hannibal and Attorney, 'How to Write a Living Will', *Www.Nolo.Com* <https://www.nolo.com/legal-encyclopedia/how-write-living-will.html> [accessed 21 November 2019].

[127] 'Power of Attorney' <https://www.americanbar.org/groups/real_property_trust_estate/resources/estate_planning/power_of_attorney/> [accessed 22 November 2019].

128 'Treatment and Management of Lewy Body Dementia', *National Institute on Aging* <https://www.nia.nih.gov/health/treatment-and-management-lewy-body-dementia> [accessed 24 April 2019].

CPSIA information can be obtained
at www.ICGtesting.com
Printed in the USA
FSHW012316171021
85534FS

9 781706 774310